Integrative Treatment of
HYPERTENSION

A Clinical and Mechanistic Approach

Integrative Treatment of
HYPERTENSION

A Clinical and Mechanistic Approach

Joel A. Blush, M.D., Ph.D.

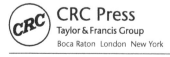

CRC Press
Taylor & Francis Group
Boca Raton London New York

CRC Press is an imprint of the
Taylor & Francis Group, an **informa** business

CRC Press
Taylor & Francis Group
6000 Broken Sound Parkway NW, Suite 300
Boca Raton, FL 33487-2742

First issued in paperback 2016

© 2014 by Taylor & Francis Group, LLC
CRC Press is an imprint of Taylor & Francis Group, an Informa business

No claim to original U.S. Government works

Version Date: 20130719

ISBN 13: 978-1-138-03411-2 (pbk)
ISBN 13: 978-1-4822-0609-8 (hbk)

Library of Congress Cataloging-in-Publication Data

Blush, Joel A., author.
  Integrative treatment of hypertension : a clinical and mechanistic approach / Joel A. Blush.
    p. ; cm.
  Includes bibliographical references and index.
  ISBN 978-1-4822-0609-8 (hardcover : alk. paper)
  I. Title.
  [DNLM: 1. Hypertension--therapy. 2. Complementary Therapies--methods. 3. Integrative Medicine--methods. WG 340]

  RC685.H8
  616.1'3206--dc23   2013028508

Visit the Taylor & Francis Web site at
http://www.taylorandfrancis.com

and the CRC Press Web site at
http://www.crcpress.com

Dedication

To Tzivie, Avi, Asher, and any new additions who come along.

Contents

Preface

The epidemic of hypertension affects about 1 billion people worldwide. In the United States alone, some 90 million people have this disease. It is a major risk factor for cardiovascular disease, stroke, and kidney disease. Although it is mostly a disease of the elderly, with current trends toward obesity, sedentary lifestyles, and poor diets, it is increasingly becoming a disease of the young too. An ever-increasing portion of medical budgets is allocated to its treatment, often making many drug companies quite profitable. Clever advertising and prudent public relations are the driving factors in the popularity of many drugs, despite the fact that most other drugs of the same class have near indistinguishable efficacy and side effects. Yet, despite the apparent popularity of many drugs, no patient really wants to take them. In fact, most patients, especially the younger ones, bargain and plead for more time or alternative treatments. Initially, medication is resisted by everyone, and for good reason, as it usually leads to many others along with dreaded side effects.

Unfortunately, most Western physicians are not trained in alternative treatments of disease. Although medical educators are beginning to address this shortcoming in their curriculum, pharmaceutical-based treatments are still the mainstay of therapy. This is the result of the major and most publicized studies being of this nature, which often are financed by the industry itself. And yet, natural remedies have been used for much longer, often having time-honored success and fewer to no side effects. Their cost is a fraction of the contemporary and competing drugs, but more important, patients gravitate to their use. People often describe natural remedies as healthier alternatives with no side effects. People seem to be empowered by their use, with a sense of taking back control of their health. It is no wonder that an increasing number of public media outlets are promoting these natural treatments. The demand is clearly there. All physicians, especially primary care doctors, are constantly challenged by their patients to provide alternative methods of treatment. Unfortunately, most do not and cannot acquiesce—not out of lack of willingness, but due to a lack of knowledge and reliable information.

Integrative Treatment of Hypertension: A Clinical and Mechanistic Approach is a book that offers an alternative approach to treating hypertension. The author is a board certified internist and nephrologist with a busy community practice as well as a Harvard trained doctor of chemistry, and therefore is in a position to integrate mainstream pharmacological medicine with alternative treatments. The author understands the needs of the medical community, both in terms of medical standards and patients' needs. Alternative treatment methods are meticulously analyzed based on data from respected medical journals to determine their efficacy. This book brings these methods into the realm of acceptance by the standards of the medical community, and provides sound mechanisms of action and practical implementation advice. Its evolution began at the behest of individual patients for alternative ways of treating hypertension and ultimately coalesced into a comprehensive book. *Integrative Treatment of Hypertension* is a unique work that fills a needed niche within the medical community and will no doubt be a welcomed companion to any health care provider.

This book has nine chapters but can be broadly divided into three sections. The first section has four chapters, which include a short introduction to hypertension, a detailed yet simple explanation of the mechanisms of blood pressure and hypertension, concise descriptions of several common causes of hypertension, and a review of standard medications used in treating hypertension and their side effects. The second section has four chapters and describes in detail alternative methods of treating hypertension. Emphasis is placed on mechanisms of action, similarities to standard medications, and practical advice on implementing these methods. This section describes dietary factors in treating hypertension, a review of several alternative yet common diets, the efficacy of nonconsumptive methods in treating hypertension, and descriptions of natural supplements in treating hypertension. The last section contains one chapter that outlines the guidelines for blood pressure goals, categorizes each method of hypertension treatment (medicines and alternative methods) into two broad groups (either anti-renin–angiotensin system or anti-salt/volume system), and suggests ways of implementing an integrative approach to hypertension treatment.

The book is directed toward the medical community, although the intelligent and interested reader will also appreciate it. Physicians, physician assistants, nurse practitioners, nurses, and medical residents will benefit from its content. Although its content is derived from mainstream and accepted medical journals, the proposed alternative treatments are by no means a substitute for standard medical practice or for common sense. As hypertension is the precursor of most cardiovascular disease, guidance from a trained health care provider is essential in its proper treatment.

Acknowledgments

The author gratefully acknowledges the contributions of Dr. Joel Neugarten, who provided sound advice throughout the process of writing this book. His guidance and teachings have always been well regarded and he has been an exemplary mentor during my training and thereafter. A special thanks to Dr. Bert Albert, who always provides thoughtful insight and advice. Thank you to Shani Stenger, for the descriptive and accurate illustrations. Last, an expression of heartfelt gratitude to my mother and father for their continued encouragement and advice. In particular to Dr. Marvin Blush, my father, who is my biggest fan, as well as my biggest fan, for always providing support, sound advice, and a unique prospective in the writing of this book and in all other matters.

Author

Joel A. Blush, M.D., Ph.D., is a practicing nephrologist and internist in a large community-based practice. He has a particular interest in the mechanisms of blood pressure regulation and in the treatment of hypertension, having academic responsibilities in teaching nephrology in affiliated university hospitals. He was awarded degrees in chemistry, achieving master's and doctorate degrees from Harvard University. He attended medical school at Albert Einstein College of Medicine followed by residency training in internal medicine at Montefiore Medical Center and fellowship training in nephrology at Albert Einstein College of Medicine. He has since been practicing as a dual board-certified nephrologist and internist. Dr. Blush is well published with many journal articles in chemistry, physics, and medicine, and has received several academic and research awards in these fields. With deference to his scientific training, he also has a strong interest in natural and alternative treatments of disease. Since his time as a medical student, he has pursued its study spending time in the Amazon rain forest taking courses in alternative medicine and botanical drug use. Dr. Blush brings to his practice a mixed scientific/medical and alternative/holistic approach to treating disease, specifically hypertension, and has successfully integrated this in the treatment of many patients.

chapter one

Diagnosis of hypertension

When first diagnosed with hypertension, people experience a mix of fear and emotion. They wonder what it means. Will they develop a stroke or heart disease? Will they be able to work and live a normal life? Will they require medication, and if so, for how long and what side effects will they experience? They have so many questions. Often they do not even understand what blood pressure is. Fortunately, there are many answers, although much remains unknown. It may be of some consolation that they are not alone. In fact, about 30% of people in the United States have hypertension. This rate is even higher in other developed countries, with over 50% of German people experiencing hypertension.[1] The possibility of developing hypertension is particularly significant in the elderly, who have about a 90% lifetime risk of manifesting it, even those free of disease at age 55.[2] So, those lucky enough to live to a ripe old age are likely to develop hypertension.

But exactly what is hypertension? Most guidelines define it as a blood pressure of ≥140/90 mm Hg. Despite this absolute definition, normal blood pressure is often defined as <120/80 mm Hg leaving an intermediate range of 120–139/80–89 mm Hg, which is not yet clearly defined. There are several well-established guidelines for the diagnosis and treatment of hypertension that do not uniformly agree on the level of blood pressure at which to initiate pharmacologic intervention. Some suggest treatment based on the risk of developing secondary diseases, such as heart disease and stroke. There are different thresholds suggested for starting medications in younger and healthier persons compared with older patients or those with other risk factors, such as diabetes or a history of smoking. Although risk stratification certainly is sensible, it can be cumbersome and confusing to both patients and physicians. The most recent guideline from the United States, published by the Joint National Committee (JNC),[3] provides the simplest scheme. Initially, healthy lifestyle changes are advocated, with medications initiated if a blood pressure <140/90 mm Hg is not achieved. The goal lowers to <130/80 mm Hg in those at high risk for cardiovascular disease such as people with diabetes, kidney disease, or heart disease. Although the JNC guideline is simple and easy to follow, the risk-stratified guidelines are superior in providing a more personalized treatment approach.

Many people wonder about the consequences of having hypertension. Does it really matter and will they become ill if their hypertension is left untreated? The answer is a clear yes, as the risk of heart disease and stroke has been shown to increase in such instances. In fact, these effects may begin at a blood pressure as low as 115/75 mm Hg, and there is a twofold increase in mortality from cardiac disease and stroke with every increase of 20/10 mm Hg.[4] Data from the Framingham study, which has followed the health of a large cohort of people over many years, clearly shows an association of cardiovascular events with blood pressure elevation even in the range of 130–139/85–89 mm Hg.[5] The next and important question is whether lowering blood pressure will reduce the risk of a subsequent cardiovascular event. People with hypertension may be otherwise predisposed to cardiovascular disease, and lowering their blood pressure might provide only limited benefit. Studies here, too, demonstrate the benefit of blood pressure lowering, although the target blood pressure is not quite as clear-cut. For example, in people with relatively few cardiovascular risk factors, a target of <140/90 mm Hg would be appropriate,[6] whereas for those at higher cardiovascular risk, reduction to <130/80 mm Hg is needed.[7]

The final question is which blood pressure medication should be prescribed. There are many classes of medicines and the best choice is often not obvious. Several large studies suggest an absolute reduction in blood pressure is the key factor in reducing cardiovascular risk, and that the specific class of blood pressure medication itself is not as significant.[8,9] However, in high-risk people such as those with diabetes, stroke, or cardiac disease, there may be compelling need for a particular class of medicine. Physicians should individualize therapy appropriately for their patients.

Measuring blood pressure

Accurate measurement is important in management of hypertension and the proper technique of blood pressure measurement is well described.[3] Mercury-type sphygmomanometers were used traditionally, but environmental concerns have led most physicians to use aneroid types. Although safer, these devices require routine maintenance and calibration, a practice that is often neglected. A care provider should have the subject sit in a chair with an armrest at the level of the heart and the subject's feet planted firmly on the ground; the patient should relax for at least 5 minutes prior to inflation of the cuff. Smoking, caffeine intake, and exercise should be avoided for at least 30 minutes prior to the exam. The room temperature should be above 12°C (54°F), as a cold environment may raise the blood pressure. The cuff should be placed using the brachial crease approach, which is just above the elbow, with the bladder length about 80% of the upper arm circumference and the width about 40% of the upper arm length. A cuff that is too small may result in an artificially elevated blood pressure reading and a cuff too large may yield a low reading. The end of the cuff should be about 3 cm (1 inch) above the elbow crease and the bell of the stethoscope should be placed over the brachial artery just below the end of the cuff. The care provider should then palpate the radial artery pulse and inflate the cuff until the pulse disappears. The cuff should then be inflated by another 20 mm Hg to ensure that the true systolic blood pressure is not missed and then slowly deflated by 2 mm Hg each second. Auscultation for the appearance and then disappearance of the Korotkoff sounds, which correspond to the systolic and diastolic blood pressure, is then performed. At least two measurements should be recorded and an average calculated.

Ambulatory blood pressure monitoring is another accepted modality to both diagnose and monitor hypertension. As these devices are expensive, and often not reimbursed by insurance companies, they are not routinely available in physician offices. Ambulatory monitoring is a better predictor of future cardiovascular events in both hypertensive[10] and non-hypertensive[11] people than office blood pressure monitoring. Typically, the blood pressure is checked for a 24-hour period, with measurements taken every 15 to 20 minutes during the day and hourly at night with multiple measurements being recorded. The main advantage of this approach is a better assessment of the blood pressure in a person's typical environment, compared with the stressful confines of a physician's office, which may itself cause the blood pressure elevation. After all, the typical daily blood pressure is what really matters. An interesting study from Italy confirms this effect,[12] reporting an initial increase in blood pressure of 22/16 mm Hg associated with a male physician conducting the exam. After 10 minutes of rest the blood pressure decreased to a plateau level but was still 12/8 mm Hg above the baseline level. When checked by a female nurse, the blood pressure also increased although by smaller amounts of 12/8 mm Hg and 1/0 mm Hg, respectively. This effect is minimized with ambulatory blood pressure monitoring. This method also differentially provides valuable information about the blood pressure during both the daytime and nighttime, which is important in the overall assessment. A 10% to 20% dip in blood pressure is expected during the nighttime, and failure to achieve this is predictive of future cardiovascular events.[13] It also provides critical information about the early morning blood pressure, which is often the highest reading of the day and most associated with cardiovascular events. The level of blood pressure associated with hypertension is lower in ambulatory monitoring, although the various major guidelines differ slightly in cutoff values. For example, the European Society of Hypertension associates hypertension with an average 24-hour blood pressure of ≥125–130/80 mm Hg,[14] whereas the JNC defines it as ≥135/85 mm Hg while awake or ≥120/75 while asleep.[3]

Home blood pressure measurement is the final monitoring modality. Commercially available devices, usually automated, are sold in most pharmacies for a modest price, allowing patients to monitor themselves by randomly measuring their blood pressure over the course of many weeks to months. Similar to ambulatory blood pressure monitoring, the results of self-monitoring show lower blood pressure readings than office measurements and also provide a better predictor of cardiovascular events than office blood pressure monitoring.[15] Aside from its cost effectiveness, home blood pressure monitoring more closely involves the individual in their care and health, making it a favored modality in many practices.

References

1. Centers for Disease Control and Prevention (CDC) National Center for Health Statistics. *National Health and Nutrition Examination Survey.* Hyattsville, MD: U.S. Department of Health and Human Services, Centers for Disease Control and Prevention; 2007.
2. Vasan RS, Beiser A, Seshadri S, et al. Residual lifetime risk for developing hypertension in middle-aged women and men. *JAMA.* 2002;287:1003–1010.
3. Chobanian AV, Bakris GL, Black HR, et al. Seventh Report of the Joint National Committee on Prevention, Detection, Evaluation, and Treatment of High Blood Pressure. *Hypertension.* 2003;42:1206–1252.
4. Prospective Studies Collaboration. Age-specific relevance of usual blood pressure to vascular mortality: A meta-analysis of individual data for one million adults in 61 prospective studies. *Lancet.* 2002;360:1903–1913.
5. Vasan RS, Larson MG, Leip EP, et al. Impact of high-normal blood pressure on the risk of cardiovascular disease. *N Eng J Med.* 2001;345:1291–1297.
6. Hansson L, Zanchetti A, Carruthers SG, et al. Effects of intensive blood-pressure lowering and low dose aspirin in patients with hypertension: Principal results of the Hypertension Optimal Treatment (HOT) randomised trial. HOT Study Group. *Lancet.* 1998;351:1755–1762.
7. Arauz-Pacheco C, Parrott MA, Raskin P, American Diabetes Association. Treatment of hypertension in adults with diabetes. *Diabetes Care.* 2003;26:S80–82.
8. Staessen JA, Wang JG, Thijs L. Cardiovascular prevention and blood pressure reduction: A quantitative overview updated until 1 March 2003. *J Hypertens.* 2003;21:1055–1076.
9. Psaty BM, Lumley T, Furberg CD, et al. Health outcomes associated with various antihypertensive therapies used as first-line agents: A network meta-analysis. *JAMA.* 2003;289:2534–2544.
10. Dolan E, Stanton A, Thijs L, et al. Superiority of ambulatory over clinic blood pressure measurement in predicting mortality: The Dublin outcome study. *Hypertension.* 2005;46:156–161.
11. Hansen TW, Jeppesen J, Rasmussen S, Ibsen H, Torp-Pedersen C. Ambulatory blood pressure and mortality: A population-based study. *Hypertension.* 2005;45:499–504.
12. Mancia G, Parati G, Pomidossi G, Grassi G, Casadei R, Zanchetti A. Alerting reaction and rise in blood pressure during measurement by physician and nurse. *Hypertension.* 1987;9:209–215.

13. Verdecchia P, Schillaci G, Gatteschi C, et al. Blunted nocturnal fall in blood pressure in hypertensive women with future cardiovascular morbid events. *Circulation*. 1993;88:986–992.

14. Mancia G, De Backer G, Dominiczak A, et al. Guidelines for management of arterial hypertension: The Task Force for the Management of Arterial Hypertension of the European Society of Hypertension (ESH) and of the European Society of Cardiology (ESC). *Eur Heart J.* 2007;28:1462–1536.

15. Ohkubo T, Imai Y, Tsuji I, et al. Home blood pressure measurement has a stronger predictive power for mortality than does screening blood pressure measurement: A population-based observation in Ohasama, Japan. *J Hypertens*. 1998;16:971–975.

chapter two

Principles of hypertension

To adequately treat hypertension, an understanding of its physical and biological mechanisms is important. When I was in medical school we were encouraged to memorize long lists of clinical symptoms and laboratory values that describe various medical illnesses; I referred to them as laundry lists. This didactic mode of study was encouraged and rewarded, but I found it did not adequately teach the principles and mechanisms of medicine. Personally, I find it difficult to remember random facts unless they are associated with a broader understanding of a process. To assist in my studies, I incorporated these random facts into models to explain medical pathology, a learning technique I still use. The study of blood pressure and hypertension is no different, and a mechanistic understanding of its principles should lead to better treatment. This chapter will describe the fundamentals of blood pressure and hypertension through basic principles of physics and biology. Although this description is not essential to using this text as a tool in treating hypertension, understanding it will facilitate its use and broaden the reader's perception of blood pressure.

The circulatory system can be described as a network of tubes or pipes connected to a pump, similar to the plumbing in a house. The pipes represent the blood vessels, the water the blood supply, and the municipal water company that pumps the water represents the heart. The water company provides the initial force, which facilitates the flow of water through the pipes. If the pumping force, that is, the water pressure, is increased, more water flows through the pipes. Similarly, if the heart pumps harder it will increase its flow, sending more blood through the blood vessels (Figure 2.1).

In physical terms, fluid flow is described by Poiseuille's law, which states that the flow of a liquid through a system is determined by the pressure within the system divided by the resistance of the system:

$$\text{Flow} = \text{Pressure/Resistance}$$

To further expand on the plumbing analogy, imagine a garden hose with a spout at its end. The initial force, or pressure, that sends water through the hose is again provided by the water company. For simplicity, we will assume it is a constant force, which is similar to the near-constant pumping force of the heart. As the water leaves the spout, its pressure is

7

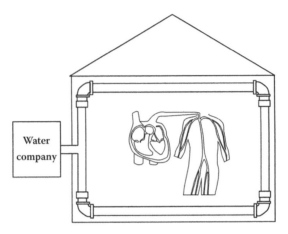

Figure 2.1 Comparison of the circulatory system with plumbing in a house. (Courtesy of Shani Strenger from Shilo, Israel.)

practically zero, so a drop in pressure must have occurred between the origin of the hose and its end. This decrease is due to the water having to work against frictional forces within the hose, or the resistance of the hose, that ultimately dissipate its force. The resistance itself is dependent on factors such as the inner diameter of the hose (or blood vessel) and the viscosity of the fluid (or blood). Of these two components, the diameter is more important, as a decrease in its size will cause an exponential increase in the resistance. Fluid viscosity is less important and often of no consequence, because the difference in viscosity of water within homes or the difference in blood viscosity from person to person is quite small. Now imagine placing your thumb over the end of the garden hose, as done when spraying water on plants (Figure 2.2). By constricting the orifice of the hose, you are decreasing the diameter of the spout, which will cause an increase in the resistance inside the hose. The total resistance is equal to the sum of the resistances of each segment. In our example, the garden hose can be divided into two parts: the long segment starting from the spigot to the thumb and the short segment of the thumb itself (Figure 2.2). The first portion, although long, has a relatively wide diameter, and therefore a minimal contribution to the total resistance. The last segment, which is only the length of your thumb, contributes much more to the total resistance because you are reducing the diameter of the hose. In fact, by placing your thumb over the spout you have created a system in which the water pressure is nearly equal throughout most of the length of the hose, but then quickly drops off at the spout. It is only in this last small segment of high resistance that the water pressure drops to zero. This example helps us to understand the circulatory system of the body. The water company represents the heart and serves to pump the fluid

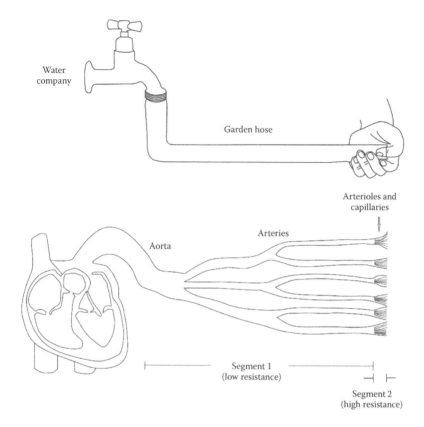

Figure 2.2 Comparison of the circulatory system with a garden hose. (Courtesy of Shani Strenger from Shilo, Israel.)

throughout the system (Figure 2.2). If the pumping activity is increased, the pressure will increase proportionately. The resistance of the blood vessels is mostly determined by the diameter of the blood vessels.

In biological terms, Poiseuille's law can be restated as:

$$CO \text{ (i.e., flow)} = \text{Blood pressure/Vascular resistance}$$

or in terms of the blood pressure:

$$\text{Blood pressure} = CO \times \text{Vascular resistance}$$

The heart initially pumps the blood to the aorta and then travels through a network of branching vessels, which get progressively smaller in diameter. Close to the end of the arterial system, there is a significant fanning out of the arterial tree into the thin-walled arterioles, which lead into the capillary plexus. The arteriolar and capillary systems are the final

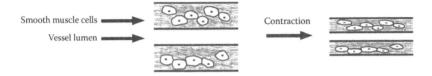

Figure 2.3 Regulation of arteriole lumen diameter by smooth muscle cells. (Courtesy of Shani Strenger from Shilo, Israel.)

segments of the arterial tree, which comprise a very short segment of the entire network and feed into the body's organs and muscles, where nutrients and oxygen are exchanged (Figure 2.2). The arterioles are very narrow vessels surrounded by a layer of smooth muscle cells, which help regulate their inner diameter (Figure 2.3). As the diameter of the arterioles are much smaller than the more proximal arteries, their contribution to the total resistance is much more significant despite their relatively short length. The short segment of arteriolar vessels can be compared to the short segment of the garden hose occluded by the thumb in the previous example. Most of the blood pressure dissipates within the arteriolar segment, which conveniently provides a near constant blood pressure to the more proximal arterial segments, such as the aorta and the small and large arteries of the arms and legs. It is important that this near-constant blood pressure (the central blood pressure) feeds the body's vital organs, including the heart, liver, kidneys, and brain. If this pressure is too low, these organs will not be adequately perfused, resulting in ischemia, heart attack, stroke, and organ malfunction. The main function of the arteriolar segment is to regulate and maintain the central blood pressure by altering the diameter of the arterioles through overlying smooth muscle contraction and dilation. In summary, the heart and the arterial system—similar to the water company and the garden hose—regulate the blood pressure in the central compartment of the body.

To illustrate this principle, imagine a person who is dehydrated, and because of a decrease in blood flow (i.e., CO) will have low blood pressure. In response to this crisis, the heart rate and contractility would increase resulting in an increase in the CO and a decrease in the arteriolar diameter causing an increase in systemic resistance and blood pressure. These compensatory mechanisms act together to help maintain an adequate blood pressure.

We now can describe several mechanisms involved in the development of hypertension. There is considerable evidence that hypertension originates with a state of high CO, and at some point transitions to a state of low or normal CO but with high vascular resistance. A long-term study of young hypertensive people who were followed over 20 years illustrates this point.[1] In youth, hypertension is driven by a state of elevated CO and normal vascular resistance. After 10 years, these indices reversed with a lower CO and higher vascular resistance. After 20 years, this pattern was even more exaggerated. To adequately appreciate this transition over time, an understanding of the role of the sympathetic nervous system in regulating blood pressure is essential.

Sympathetic nervous system and blood pressure

The brain has several centers that regulate the function of other organs such as the heart, blood vessels, kidneys, and adrenal glands. Activity in these centers is increased during states of emotional or physical excitement. A common laboratory model of induced stress involves a person attempting to solve a difficult math problem. The fight-or-flight response is another example of a sudden frightful stimulus activating these centers with a resultant increase in heart rate and blood pressure. The nerve cells end in synapses at their target organs where they release norepinephrine, thereby signaling for an increase in blood pressure (Figure 2.4). Norepinephrine stimulates the beta-receptors of the heart causing it to beat more quickly and forcefully, increasing the CO and, consequently, the blood pressure. The alpha-receptors of the blood vessels also are activated, causing vasoconstriction and subsequent increases in both resistance and blood pressure. Simultaneous activation of the kidney beta-receptors stimulates the renin–angiotensin–aldosterone system (RAAS), another important component in blood pressure regulation. This activation also causes the kidneys to retain salt and water, with a further increase in CO and blood pressure. Last, the sympathetic nervous system stimulates the adrenal glands to produce yet more systemic norepinephrine.

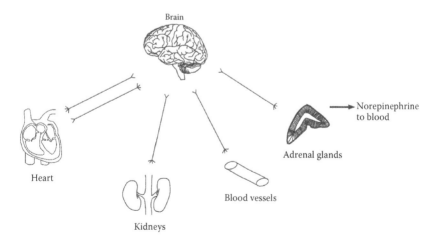

Figure 2.4 Regulation of body organ function by the sympathetic nervous system. (Courtesy of Shani Strenger from Shilo, Israel.)

The regulatory centers of the brain receive signals from a variety of sources, including other brain areas, pressure and chemical sensors in the heart (left ventricle and left atrium), and the great outlet vessels of the heart (aortic arch and carotid sinus). The sensors help attenuate low blood pressure, as may occur in dehydration, by sending stimulatory signals to the brain. Pain and emotional stress also stimulate these centers.

There is considerable evidence that young people with hypertension have an overactive sympathetic nervous system referred to as a hyperkinetic state.[2] This was demonstrated in a study finding elevated norepinephrine levels in young hypertensive people compared with age-matched subjects with normal blood pressure.[3] Younger people also tend to have higher heart rates and an elevated CO compared with older people with hypertension. However, with age, the hypertension transitions to increased vascular resistance and relatively normal CO. Although some suggest this is due to a shift to a state of lower sympathetic activity, it has been found that sympathetic nervous system activity actually increases as people age.[4] Plasma norepinephrine levels in people with normal blood pressure have been shown to increase with age until they eventually reach the levels of young people with hypertension, and typical norepinephrine levels in elderly people with hypertension are similar to age-matched nonhypertensive people.[3] Julius and Nesbitt[2] present an interesting theory to explain this transition and potentially the root cause of hypertension. They suggest that the brains of people with hypertension reset to a higher blood pressure norm. In young people, the heart is very responsive to norepinephrine and is able to maintain a higher blood pressure by increasing the CO. However, as people age, the cardiac receptors become less responsive to norepinephrine, and the ability of the heart to contract also diminishes precluding its ability to increase blood flow and pressure. This is probably due to fibrosis and thickening of the heart wall. However, with age and chronically elevated blood pressure, the muscular wall surrounding the blood vessels undergoes hypertrophy, thus increasing its ability to contract when stimulated by norepinephrine. These vessels constrict in response to relatively lower levels of norepinephrine causing an increase in vascular resistance and subsequent hypertension. This provides a reasonable explanation of the aging transition in hypertension. Although a resetting of nervous system activity may cause hypertension, it is still unclear what prompts this process as that only would be the true etiology of hypertension.

Arterial stiffness and endothelial dysfunction

Based on the relative diameter size of the blood vessels, the arterial system can be divided into two parts: (1) the aorta and arteries, and (2) the arterioles and capillaries (Figure 2.5). As previously described, there is a

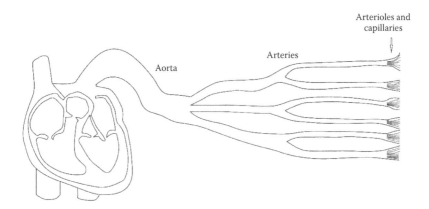

Figure 2.5 Schematic of the arterial tree. (Courtesy of Shani Strenger from Shilo, Israel.)

sudden transition to higher vessel resistance when moving from the aorta and arteries to the arterioles and capillaries. This is due to the significant decrease in the diameter of the vessel lumen, as resistance increases exponentially with smaller lumen sizes. A typical artery has a lumen of about 0.5 cm (0.2 inch), whereas an arteriole lumen is about 1/1000th this size. There is also a dramatic branching pattern that occurs at the interface of the arteries and arterioles.

The structure of the vessel walls of these two systems also is different. The walls of the aorta and arteries are mainly composed of elastin and collagen, which gives them a rubbery or elastic property. In contrast, the arteriole walls are composed of smooth muscle cells and are more rigid with the ability to constrict and dilate. As the heart pumps blood into the aorta and arteries, the elasticity of these vessels buffers the forceful pulse and slows its flow. Imagine our previous image of a water faucet connected to a rubber hose. When the faucet is suddenly opened, the water rushes into the hose. If the hose is rubbery, it will expand as the pulse of water travels through it, thus slowing the flow of water and reducing the pressure. A normal and healthy aorta serves the same purpose by buffering the high-pressure pulse with each heartbeat and slowing its flow. As the pulse reaches the arteriolar system, it abruptly contacts stiffer vessels of higher resistance and multiple branching points as the arteriolar system fans out. This dramatic change in resistance, stiffness, and branching causes a part of the pulse to be reflected backward toward the aorta.[5] This effect is similar to an echo produced when calling out hello at the foot of a canyon (Figure 2.6). As the pressure packet of the sound wave reaches the opposing wall of the canyon, it is reflected back, and a few seconds later the same hello echoes back, although softer.

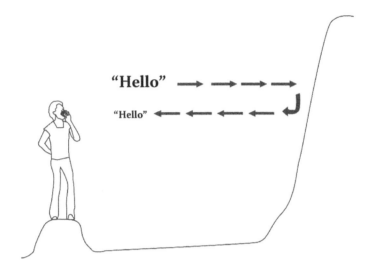

Figure 2.6 Schematic of reflected sound wave packet. (Courtesy of Shani Strenger from Shilo, Israel.)

Now imagine saying "hello, hello, hello" but spacing the words with enough time for the echoes to return between each spoken hello. You would hear a continuous succession of six hellos despite only uttering three. The three uttered hellos would be louder than the three echoed hellos (Figure 2.7a). Now compare this image to the pulse of blood created with each heartbeat. Each uttered hello is analogous to a contraction of the heart and its subsequent pulse of blood, which is the systolic phase of blood flow. The time between the three uttered hellos is analogous to the period that the heart muscle relaxes and fills with blood, that is, the diastolic phase of blood flow. As the blood pulse travels through the aorta and arteries it is first slowed by their elasticity. When it reaches the arteriolar segment, a part of the pulse is reflected back through the same vessels toward the heart in a manner similar to the echoed hellos in the canyon (Figure 2.7b).

In a healthy vascular system this reflected wave slowly returns to the arteries and the aorta during the quiescent (diastolic) phase of the cardiac cycle (Figure 2.8a). This helps to buffer the blood pressure during a time in the cycle that it would normally be low. Because the diastolic phase comprises about two-thirds of the cardiac cycle, it is important to sustain an adequate pressure during this period to properly perfuse the body organs. The timing of this reflected pulse varies according to the elasticity of the aorta and the arteries, and the stiffness and degree of branching of the arterioles. If the larger blood vessels are stiff (i.e., nonelastic) or if the arteriolar resistance is large, then the reflected wave will return quickly and encroach on the systolic phase of the cycle. This will cause an elevated

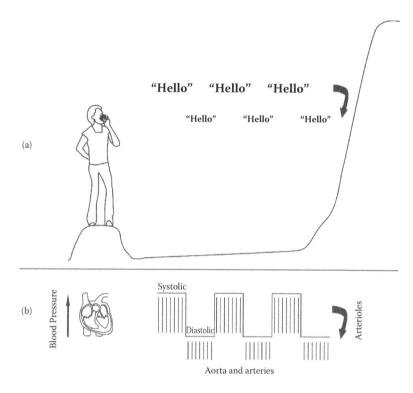

Figure 2.7 Comparison of reflected sound wave packet with reflected blood pressure pulse/packet. (Courtesy of Shani Strenger from Shilo, Israel.)

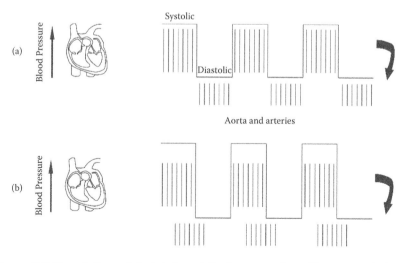

Figure 2.8 Description of isolated systolic hypertension. (Courtesy of Shani Strenger from Shilo, Israel.)

systolic blood pressure and a lower diastolic blood pressure, a condition referred to as isolated systolic hypertension, which is a marker of vascular disease (Figure 2.8b). The condition exerts strain on the heart as it has to pump into a system of higher pressure, and is associated with accelerated atherosclerosis and cardiovascular disease. Isolated systolic hypertension is more common in the elderly, in people with diabetes, and in those with vascular disease.

An understanding of arterial stiffness will help to better appreciate this concept. Arterial stiffness can be explained by three structural and functional characteristics: remodeling of the vessels, endothelial dysfunction, and atherosclerosis. Although each of these characteristics can be considered distinct processes, they are actually all interrelated and better thought of as a continuum. Although convenient to describe the arterial system as a set of pipes or conduits that transport the blood from the heart to the organs, this is a gross oversimplification. In fact, the circulatory system is a vibrant and adaptable organ. Vessel walls are composed of an inner single layer of endothelial cells surrounded by a mesh of smooth muscle cells. The matrix that holds them together is composed of collagen and elastin (Figure 2.9). Although the endothelium is only one cell thick, it is so expansive that it covers over 1300 square meters (14000 square feet) of surface area (a mansion by any standard) and weighs up to 3 kilograms (6–7 pounds).[6] It is the largest organ in the body. The endothelium acts as the interface between the blood and the vessel wall, and helps to regulate vessel tone and size. It senses changes within the circulatory system, such as higher blood pressure or bloodborne chemical/humoral agents, and transmits signals to the overlying smooth muscle cells and matrix. These signals regulate the vessel tone. The system is very complex and involves many chemical messengers, but can be characterized by two distinct and opposite states: either upregulated/activated or quiescent/inactivated. The former state occurs in disease when humoral signals cause the vessels to constrict; this state promotes atherosclerosis

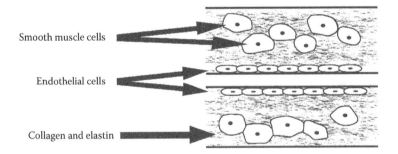

Smooth muscle cells

Endothelial cells

Collagen and elastin

Figure 2.9 Structure of the arteriole wall. (Courtesy of Shani Strenger from Shilo, Israel.)

and scar tissue deposition and is referred to as endothelial dysfunction. The inactivated state occurs in health; it is quiescent when the vessels are appropriately dilated and there is minimal atherosclerotic deposition. In the healthy endothelium, there is a favorable balance toward the quiescent/inactivated state despite the presence of minimal stresses or activating chemical messengers. However, when the endothelium is injured or dysfunctional, the balance is quickly tipped toward the activated state. Endothelial dysfunction is strongly associated with atherosclerosis, hypertension, and cardiovascular disease. It is also associated with smoking,[7] elevated cholesterol levels,[8] obesity, diabetes,[9] and a sedentary lifestyle.[10] Two important chemical messengers that regulate the endothelium are angiotensin II and nitric oxide, which may serve as representatives of the larger group of chemicals within each class. Angiotensin II is associated with vasoconstriction, atherosclerosis, and hypertension, whereas nitric oxide (perhaps its nemesis) is associated with vasodilation, reduced atherosclerosis, and normal blood pressure. Endothelial function has important effects on arterial stiffness. In states of endothelial dysfunction the large arterial vessels are stiffer and the resistance within the arterioles is higher. Consequently, the pulse wave of the blood is reflected backward more rapidly and forcefully, resulting in systolic hypertension and often isolated systolic hypertension.

Renin–angiotensin–aldosterone system

The renin–angiotensin–aldosterone system (RAAS) is an essential part of blood pressure regulation. It is a complex system involving several enzymes, substrates, chemical messengers, and organs (Figure 2.10). An appreciation of RAAS mechanics is essential to understanding blood pressure regulation and the proper choice of antihypertensive therapy. The first substance in this system is angiotensinogen, produced in the liver. It is a relatively stable molecule with a long half-life and its biological

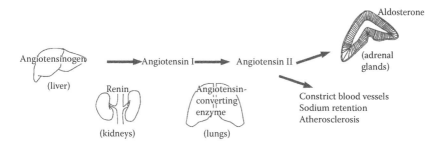

Figure 2.10 The renin–angiotensin–aldosterone system. (Courtesy of Shani Strenger from Shilo, Israel.)

function is rather limited as a substrate of the enzyme renin, which converts it to angiotensin I. Renin is primarily produced by the kidneys and circulates in the bloodstream. As the conversion of angiotensinogen to angiotensin I is the rate-limiting step of the RAAS, the activity of renin importantly regulates the entire system. Angiotensin I also has limited biologic function but is converted to angiotensin II, which has prominent biological effects causing constriction of blood vessels, sodium and water retention by the kidneys, and atherosclerotic changes to the vessels, all of which promote elevated blood pressure. The conversion is catalyzed by angiotensin-converting enzyme, which is mostly produced in the lungs. Angiotensin II also stimulates the adrenal glands to produce aldosterone, which also has many biological functions. Aldosterone promotes salt and water retention by the kidneys, and elevated levels are associated with cardiovascular events such as stroke and heart attack.[11] Because it involves several distinct organs, the RAAS is classically described as a systemic system. However, there is also an independent system that is local to all tissue, referred to as the local RAAS, which is particularly important to the heart and blood vessels.

The kidneys have a key role in the RAAS and blood pressure regulation. These organs primarily filter the blood, and as much as 25% of the entire blood flow typically passes through them, amounting to some 180 liters of filtered plasma each day. If not for its ability to reabsorb most of the filtrate (over 99%) we would quickly dehydrate. This delicate process enables the kidneys to maintain the body's balance of electrolytes and fluid. The functional unit of the kidney is the nephron, and each kidney contains about one million of them. Each nephron is a distinct unit that manages a tiny fraction of filtrate (or urine), but collectively they manage the entire process. It is also important in regulating production of the enzyme renin. The nephron is composed of the renal corpuscle and the renal tubule (Figure 2.11). The renal corpuscle is a ball-like microscopic structure composed of a matrix of interweaving capillaries known as the glomerulus, and a surrounding structure called the Bowman's capsule. The capillaries of glomerulus are fed by the afferent arteriole and drained by the efferent arteriole. Filtration occurs within the glomerulus, and the filtrate is collected into Bowman's capsule, which leads into the first segment of the renal tubule. The tubule is a winding conduit where most of the electrolytes and water are reabsorbed back into the bloodstream leaving mostly toxic waste for disposal in the urine. As a part of the winding pathway, the tubule circles back and contacts the afferent arteriole just adjacent to the glomerulus. This area of contact (the juxtaglomerular apparatus) is the region where renin is produced and secreted. The apparatus is strategically located so it can receive information about the blood pressure via the pressure within the afferent arteriole, and about the fluid balance of the body from the chemical composition of the tubule filtrate.

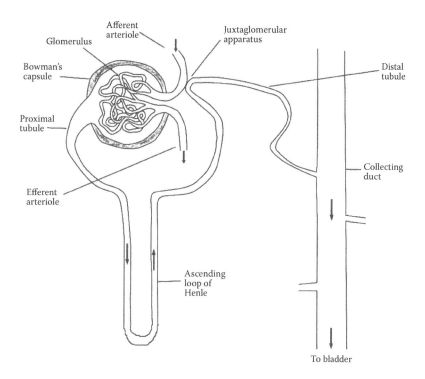

Figure 2.11 Schematic of the nephron. (Courtesy of Shani Strenger from Shilo, Israel.)

It also receives direct input from the central nervous system via nerve endings. All of these inputs importantly regulate renin production and subsequently the RAAS. For example, in a state of dehydration, the kidney's nephrons will sense a low blood pressure and a concentrated tubular filtrate, which will enhance renin production and the RAAS. Because it receives input directly from the central nervous system, it can also be activated by heightened sympathetic nervous system activity such as what happens in frightening or emotional situations. The RAAS is of particular importance in treatment of hypertension as several classes of medicines block different parts of its pathway.

Salt sensitivity

The influence of salt on blood pressure has been known for millennia. Texts of the Chinese emperor Haung Ti over 4000 years ago describe a relationship between salt intake and a "hardened pulse," a reference to hypertension. Our genetic makeup is structured to preserve salt and water in order to maintain an adequate blood pressure. Imagine the struggled survival of prehistoric man with a meager supply of food and water. Salt was a rare commodity in the late Paleolithic period (some 10,000 years ago), with a diet consisting mostly of fruits, nuts, legumes, and some animal products and a sodium intake of about only 600 mg (26 meq) a day.[12] In comparison, a typical Western diet consists of over 3000 mg (130 meq) of sodium a day[13] with over 75% coming from nondiscretionary sources such as added preservatives and flavor enhancers. There appears to be a set point between 1150 and 2300 mg (50–100 meq) of daily sodium intake at which salt-mediated hypertension manifests.[14] Ironically, the recommended daily intake is up to 2300 mg (100 meq or 1 teaspoon of salt).[15] Our prehistoric genome, which is probably similar to that of today, is geared to preserve sodium, which was essential to properly subsist in prehistoric times but not in modern times. However, such cultures still exist, as evident in the Yanomamo Indians of the Amazon rain forest, who have a typical sodium intake of only about 25 mg (1 meq) a day.[16] Not surprisingly, there is no hypertension in this society, which has a typical blood pressure of only 100/65 mm Hg. Ironically, our adaptive quality of conserving sodium to preserve blood pressure is now a cause of hypertension and pathology. Many have studied the effects of sodium intake on blood pressure. Although some studies demonstrate large differences in blood pressure between low and high sodium diets, the generally accepted value is a modest difference of only 3 to 5/2 mm Hg. In terms of an entire population, lowering of blood pressure by this amount would have a great impact on public health, although the effect would be minimal to the individual with hypertension. Yet, despite the clear association of elevated sodium intake and hypertension, it is not clear that excessive sodium intake increases the risk of adverse effects, specifically heart disease, stroke, and kidney disease in people with hypertension. In fact, some report fewer adverse outcomes in people with and without hypertension who consume higher amounts of sodium.[17,18]

The effects of sodium intake on health will be discussed in a later chapter, but a description of its effect on blood pressure will now be presented. The primary effect of salt (or sodium) intake on blood pressure is to increase the volume of the plasma component of blood, which results in an increase in CO and blood pressure. Its secondary effect is from the vascular response to this increased flow, which results in constriction of the peripheral arteriolar blood vessels, causing increased peripheral vascular resistance and blood pressure. Both of these effects raise the blood pressure as described by the equation from Poiseuille's law, which equates blood pressure with the product of cardiac output and peripheral vascular resistance (BP = CO × PVR). The kidneys have a central role in maintaining salt and water balance, and therefore they regulate salt sensitivity. The work of Guyton describes the role of the kidneys in this process.[19] From computer-generated models of hypertension he determined that the kidneys are the primary and ultimate regulator of blood pressure. He argues that every person has a blood pressure set point that is fixed by the ability of the kidneys to either retain or eliminate salt and water. This set point is pathologically elevated in people with hypertension. Various humoral factors such as angiotensin II also can influence this set point and cause elevated blood pressure. There are several prominent theories posed about the cause of salt sensitivity (Figure 2.12). Brenner suggests that hypertension may be due to a reduced nephron/glomeruli count in the kidneys.[20] Each kidney typically contains about 1 million nephrons, although this number can vary from 200,000 to 2,000,000.[21] He suggests that people with reduced nephron counts are more susceptible to hypertension because their kidneys have a limited ability to excrete sodium and water. Furthermore, from consequent adaptation of a reduced nephron count, each nephron increases its filtration capacity causing excessive pressure and strain on the entire network of glomeruli and tubules over time. The resulting scarring of the glomerus/nephron will further reduce the ability of the kidneys to excrete sodium and water. Evidence to support this theory comes from an association of a low birth weight (associated with lower nephron counts) with subsequent hypertension in adult life.[22] Further evidence is presented in a postmortem study of 20 people of similar age and race of whom 10 had hypertension and 10 had normal blood pressure. The average nephron count of the hypertensive group was about half that of the normal blood pressure group (700,000 versus 1,400,000 nephrons per kidney).[23]

Another prominent theory of salt sensitivity is proposed by Sealy and colleagues, and involves an aberrant group of nephrons that inappropriately secrete renin-causing activation of the RAAS.[24] The primary stimulus of secretory activity comes from blood pressure sensors in the walls of the arterioles that lead into the glomerulus, that is, the afferent arterioles (Figure 2.11). In response to low blood pressure, the nephron will secrete more renin and activate the RAAS to raise the blood pressure. In normal health, when all the blood vessels are patent and connected in an open and free flowing way, the pressure in the arterioles reflects the pressure throughout the body. However, if a group of these arterioles is clogged or blocked (i.e., ischemia), they will have a reduced pressure within them despite a normal overall blood pressure in the rest of the body. These aberrant nephrons will secrete renin despite normal or even elevated blood pressure in the body. Because there are only a few of these nephrons, their contribution to the overall body renin level is diluted and usually results in a small increase. However, even a small amount of renin is abnormal in hypertension and is sufficient to cause the other normal nephrons to retain more salt and water, further increasing the blood pressure. This theory explains why renin levels are often present in people with elevated blood pressure when the RAAS ideally should be completely shut down.

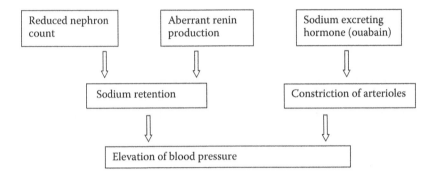

Figure 2.12 Mechanism of salt sensitivity.

The last theory of salt sensitivity is more complex and as yet not fully developed. Its contributions span many decades and involve the works of several scientists.[25–27] In states of volume excess, as after eating a large meal with salt and fluid, a "sodium excreting hormone" is produced. By inactivating sodium–potassium pumps found in the nephron tubules, this hormone facilitates purging the body of excess salt and water. However, this hormone also inactivates the sodium–potassium pumps of the smooth muscle cells of the arterioles (Figure 2.3). This causes excessive calcium influx into the smooth muscle cells and leads to contraction of these cells and constriction of the arteriolar vessels and a consequent increase in peripheral vascular resistance and blood pressure. Overall, this theory proposes that an increase in salt intake will lead to production of a humoral substance that will cause constriction of the blood vessels and hypertension. Some feel that this humoral substance is a protein called ouabain,[28] although this has not been conclusively proven. Although these three popular mechanisms of salt sensitivity are well known, many other theories exist. It is likely that there is no single unifying cause of salt sensitivity and hypertension but rather that each person has his or her own specific cause. Nonetheless, the treatment is the same and requires salt reduction and diuretic therapy.

Renin profiling

The enzyme renin regulates the activity of the entire RAAS. Although considered to have few direct biological effects, a limited role in causing vascular inflammation and scarring is suggested by recent studies. However, its main function is to convert angiotensinogen to angiotensin I, a process that regulates the entire RAAS through the production of the active agents angiotensin II and aldosterone. Laragh and colleagues have elegantly characterized the role of the RAAS in blood pressure control. Their contribution to the study and understanding of hypertension cannot be overstated. They describe human blood pressure in terms of two supporting systems: the salt/volume system and the RAAS. Under normal conditions, blood pressure is supported by the quantity of salt and water in the body. Salt, particularly sodium, causes an increase in blood volume, thus increasing the CO component of blood pressure. It also causes a secondary constriction of the arteriolar vessels, increasing the peripheral vascular resistance and supporting blood pressure. When blood volume is decreased, for example, from dehydration (a lack of salt and water) or poor heart function (heart failure), the RAAS is activated as a backup system to support blood pressure. Although the primary function of this system is to constrict the peripheral vessels, it also stimulates the kidneys to retain salt and water. In a healthy person without hypertension, these systems act together to maintain a normal blood pressure. When salt and water are appropriately balanced, the RAAS is turned off. Similarly, it is turned off in states of excess salt and water, thus allowing the kidneys to rid the body of these elements and return the blood pressure to normal. Hypertension is a pathologic state in which the body either retains salt and water, or activates the RAAS; often both processes are activated. Laragh characterizes these two forms of hypertension as either V (volume/salt-mediated) type or R (renin) type. Most people have a combination of both contributing to their hypertension. He also classifies blood pressure medications in terms of either V- or R-type, depending on which axis they primarily affect. After decades of clinical and scientific study he formulated the Laragh method,[29,30] which uses the plasma renin activity (PRA) to guide treatment of hypertension. For example, if a person with hypertension has a low PRA the cause is likely excess salt/volume and a diuretic would be the appropriate initial medication to prescribe. If hypertension persists despite an adequate diuretic dose, the PRA can be repeated to further guide treatment. This technique is referred to as renin profiling. It adds a logical and scientific rationale to the treatment of hypertension and should facilitate therapy with the use of fewer medications. As natural medicines and techniques have generally been poorly characterized clinically or experimentally, the V- and R-type classification also can be used to define their properties allowing a scientific basis for their use. This book will attempt to characterize all forms of blood pressure lowering methods, which include traditional medicines, natural medicines, and various techniques, according to their ability to modify these two axes of blood pressure regulation. This system of classification allows for an integrated approach to managing hypertension, using all forms of antihypertensive therapeutic modalities.

Despite the simplicity and elegance of the Laragh method, there are skeptics. Large studies of randomly treated people with hypertension have found specific drug classes more potent in certain age and race groups. For example, calcium channel blockers are more effective in black men, whereas angiotensin-converting enzyme inhibitors have been shown to be superior in young white men.[31] This age and race profiling has been suggested by some to be a better predictor of medication response.[32] Nonetheless, the elegant and simple renin profiling technique is a powerful and effective tool.

References

1. Lund-Johansen P. Central haemodynamics in essential hypertension at rest and during exercise: A 20-year follow-up study. *J Hypertens Suppl.* 1989;7:s52–55.
2. Julius S, Nesbitt S. Sympathetic overactivity in hypertension: A moving target. *Am J Hypertens.* 1996;9:113s–120s.
3. Goldstein DS, Lake CR, Chernow B. Age-dependence of hypertensive-normotensive differences in plasma norepinephrine. *Hypertension.* 1983;5:100–104.
4. Narkiewicz K, Phillips BG, Kato M, Hering D, Bieniaszewski L, Somers VK. Gender-selective interaction between aging, blood pressure and sympathetic nerve activity. *Hypertension.* 2005;45:522–525.
5. Mitchell GF. Arterial stiffness and wave reflection in hypertension: Pathophysiologic and therapeutic implications. *Curr Hypertens Rep.* 2004;6:436–441.
6. Halcox JPJ, Quyyumi AA. Endothelial function and cardiovascular disease. In: Izzo JL, Sica DA, Black HR, eds. *Hypertension Primer: The Essentials of High Blood Pressure*, 4th ed. Philadelphia: Lippincott Williams & Wilkins; 2008:204–208.
7. Oida K, Ebata K, Kanehara H, Suzuki J, Miyamori I. Effect of cilostazol on impaired vasodilatory response of the brachial artery to ischemia in smokers. *J Atheroscler Thromb.* 2003;10:93–98.
8. Engler MM, Engler MB, Malloy MJ, et al. Antioxidant vitamins C and E improve endothelial function in children with hyperlipidemia: Endothelial Assessment of Risk from Lipids in Youth (EARLY) Trial. *Circulation.* 2003;108:1059–1063.
9. Calles-Escandon J, Cipolla M. Diabetes and endothelial dysfunction: A clinical perspective. *Endocrine Rev.* 2001;22:36–52.
10. Green DJ, Walsh JH, Maiorana A, Best MJ, Taylor RR, O'Driscoll JG. Exercise-induced improvement in endothelial dysfunction is not mediated by changes in CV risk factors: Pooled analysis of diverse patient populations. *Am J Physiol Heart Circ Physiol.* 2003;285:H2679–2687.
11. Milliez P, Girerd X, Plouin PF, Blacher J, Safar ME, Mourad JJ. Evidence for an increased rate of cardiovascular events in patients with primary aldosteronism. *J Am Coll Cardiol.* 2005;45:1243–1248.
12. Eaton SB, Eaton SB 3rd, Konner MJ, Shostak M. An evolutionary perspective enhances understanding of human nutritional requirements. *J Nutr.* 1996;126:1732–1740.
13. Engstrom A, Tobelmann RC, Albertson AM. Sodium intake trends and food choices. *Am J Clin Nutr.* 1997;65(suppl):704s–707s.
14. Kaplan NM. Dietary salt intake and blood pressure. *JAMA.* 1984;251:1429–1430.

15. Recommendations of U.S. Department of Health and Human Services and U.S. Department of Agriculture, www.usda.gov.
16. Oliver W, Cohen EL, Neel JV. Blood pressure, sodium intake and sodium related hormones in the Yanomamo Indians, a "no-salt" culture. *Circulation.* 1975;52:146–151.
17. Alderman MH, Madhavan S, Cohen H, Sealey JE, Laragh JH. Low urinary sodium is associated with greater risk of myocardial infarction among treated hypertensive men. *Hypertension.* 1995;25:1144–1152.
18. Alderman MH, Cohen H, Madhavan S. Dietary sodium intake and mortality: The National Health and Nutrition Examination Survey (NHANES I). *Lancet.* 1998;351:781–785.
19. Guyton AC. Kidneys and fluids in pressure regulation: Small volume but large pressure changes. *Hypertension.* 1992;19(suppl I):I2–I8.
20. Brenner B, Garcia DL, Anderson S. Glomeruli and blood pressure: Less of one, more the other. *Am J Hypertens.* 1988;1:335–347.
21. Douglas-Denton RN, McNamara BJ, Hoy WE, Hughson MD, Bertram JF. Does nephron number matter in the development of kidney disease? *Ethn Dis.* 2006;16(2 suppl 2):S2-40–45.
22. Brenner B, Chertow G. Congenital oligonephropathy and the etiology of adult hypertension and progressive renal injury. *Am J Kidney Dis.* 1994;23:171–175.
23. Keller G, Zimmer G, Mall G, Ritz E, Amann K. Nephron number in patients with primary hypertension. *N Engl J Med.* 2003;348:101–108.
24. Sealy JE, Blumenfeld JD, Bell GM, Pecker MS, Sommers SC, Laragh JH. On the renal basis for essential hypertension: Nephron heterogeneity with discordant renin secretion and sodium excretion causing hypertensive vasoconstriction-volume relationship. *J Hypertens.* 1988;6:763–777.
25. Dahl LK, Knudsen KD, Iwai J. Humoral transmission of hypertension: Evidence from parabiosis. *Circ Res.* 1969;24(suppl):21–33.
26. Blaustein MP. Sodium ions, calcium ions, blood pressure regulation and hypertension: A reassessment and a hypothesis. *Am J Physiol.* 1977;232:C165–173.
27. De Wardener HE, MacGregor GA. Dahl's hypothesis that a saluretic substance may be responsible for a sustained rise in arterial pressure: Its possible role in essential hypertension. *Kidney Int.* 1980;18:1–9.
28. Iwamoto T, Kita S, Zhang J, et al. Salt-sensitive hypertension is triggered by Ca2+ entry via Na+/Ca2+ exchanger type-1 in vascular smooth muscle. *Nat Med.* 2004;10:1193–1199.
29. Laragh JH, Sealey JE. The plasma renin test reveals the contribution of body sodium-volume content (V) and renin–angiotensin (R) vasoconstriction to long-term blood pressure. *Am J Hypertens.* 2011;24:1164–1180.
30. Laragh J. Laragh's lessons in pathophysiology and clinical pearls for treating hypertension. *Am J Hypertens.* 2001;14:491–503.
31. Materson BJ, Reda DJ, Cushman WC, et al. Single-drug therapy for hypertension in men. A comparison of six antihypertensive agents with placebo. *N Engl J Med.* 1993;328:914–921.
32. Preston RA, Materson BJ, Reda DJ, et al. Age-race subgroup compared with renin profile as predictors of blood pressure response to antihypertensive therapy. *JAMA.* 1998;280:1168–1172.

chapter three

Common causes of hypertension

Stress, white-coat hypertension, and white-coat effect

Emotional and physical stress is a common entity with associated health effects, specifically in causing hypertension and cardiovascular disease. An interesting study that illustrates this compares the health of nuns in a secluded order with that of women in their local community. Lower blood pressure and decreased incidence of cardiovascular disease in the secluded nuns was noted,[1] likely in part due to their comparatively peaceful lifestyle. Another study showed blood pressure in four population centers in the United States to be significantly elevated in the months following the 9/11 terrorist attacks,[2] again an effect associated with heightened anxiety and stress. Job strain[3] and a sense of time urgency and hostility[4] also have been associated with the development of hypertension and cardiovascular disease. The mechanism whereby stress causes hypertension is primarily due to enhancement of the sympathetic nervous system, although activation of the renin–angiotensin–aldosterone system (RAAS),[5] salt retention,[6] and endothelial dysfunction[7] also occur. The degree of responsiveness to an acute stressor is also an important factor. Responsivity to stress is measured by the degree of blood pressure and heart rate increase, and the amount of time needed for these parameters to return to their respective baselines. Prolonged responsivity is strongly associated with future development of hypertension.[8] Stress responsivity is also associated with white-coat effect and white-coat hypertension.[9] The definition of white-coat effect is an increase in blood pressure that occurs during an exam by a physician—hence the term "white coat"—that can manifest in people with or without hypertension, whereas white-coat hypertension is defined as an elevated office blood pressure but a normal 24-hour ambulatory or home blood pressure. The precise definition of white-coat hypertension differs slightly depending on the guideline. For example, the European Society of Hypertension requires an office blood pressure of 140/90 mm Hg or greater, a normal 24-hour mean ambulatory blood pressure of <125–130/80 mm Hg, and a normal mean daytime blood pressure of <130–135/85 mm Hg.[10] A normal mean home blood pressure of <135/85 mm Hg also can be used. White-coat effect is nicely illustrated in an Italian study that showed an increase in blood pressure of 22/16 mm Hg when initially measured by a male physician.[11] After 10 minutes, repeat blood pressure decreased to a plateau level but was still 12/8 mmHg above baseline. White-coat hypertension is more prevalent in certain populations, occurring in 38% of Finnish hypertensive people,[12] whereas 20% is typical in Western society.[13] As many studies suggest only a minimal increase in cardiovascular risk from white-coat hypertension,[14] most guidelines do not recommend treatment with drug therapy unless there is evidence of organ damage or other significant cardiovascular risk factors. Lifestyle changes such as a low-salt diet and weight loss are recommended first. However, there is evidence suggesting a less benign nature as white-coat hypertension may be associated with cardiac hypertrophy,[15] cardiovascular disease,[16] and stroke.[17] There also is a significant risk of progressing from white-coat hypertension to overt hypertension.[18] Perhaps, it is best to view white-coat hypertension as an intermediate hypertensive state that needs careful monitoring.

Oral contraceptives

Oral contraceptives have been a popular means of birth control since the 1960s. In 2007, approximately 94 million women of reproductive age used them.[19] In 2002 in the United States alone, 11.6 million women of reproductive age were taking oral contraceptives and 82% of all women had taken them at some time in their lives,[20] representing a significant segment of the populations of both Western and developing countries. The active pharmacologic components of these medications are derivatives of the female sex hormones, estrogen, and progestin. Early formulations contained high doses of estrogen but more recently lower doses are used. Heart attack and stroke are two important and serious associations, more common with the older formulations of higher estrogen doses. Yet, even with the newer drugs that contain relatively low doses of estrogen there still is an increased risk, although lower, of developing heart attack[21] or stroke.[22] However, as these events are quite infrequent in young women of reproductive age, the total overall number of such events is very low. Furthermore, most complications occur in either smokers or women with hypertension, leaving the more typical and healthy women with no appreciably increased risk. The American College of Obstetricians and Gynecologists support oral contraceptive use by women of all ages, except for those over 35 years who smoke.[23] It suggests caution in women with hypertension but still support its use with careful blood pressure monitoring. The estrogen component is the cause of increase in blood pressure, despite its known vasodilatory effect. Activation of the RAAS may be a contributing factor.[24] In women with normal blood pressure, an increase of 8/6 mm Hg on 24-hour ambulatory blood pressure monitoring is expected,[25] and up to 5% of women with normal blood pressure may reach levels of hypertension.[26] Malignant hypertension is also reported, although a rare event. Physicians should carefully monitor their patients who are taking these medications. Fortunately, the blood pressure returns to its prior level when the medication is stopped.

Obstructive sleep apnea

Obstructive sleep apnea (OSA) is a common respiratory ailment caused by intermittent airway collapse during sleep. Pauses in breathing cause disruption of sleep and episodes of decreased blood oxygen levels. This may occur in as much as 20% of people in Western society.[27] People with OSA experience fatigue throughout the day, are prone to motor vehicle accidents, and have psychosocial problems and decreased cognitive function. OSA is also associated with hypertension,[28] cardiovascular disease, and stroke. Although obesity is the classic risk factor for its development, it is also more common in smokers, males, and the elderly. In healthy people a dip in blood pressure typically occurs overnight, but this is often absent in people with OSA, with blood pressure increases more common. There is a strong association with sudden cardiac death during sleep, a time that is otherwise protective of such events.[29] Stimulation of brain centers causing increased sympathetic neural activity is the most important contributing factor to increased blood pressure,[30] although increased levels of angiotensin II[31] and aldosterone,[32] and endothelial dysfunction[33] also occur. Ideally, OSA can be treated through lifestyle changes such as weight loss, smoking cessation, and exercise, but often requires continuous positive airway pressure (CPAP) throughout the night to keep from airway collapse. Blood pressure may decrease with CPAP therapy.[34] Although this is a cumbersome and noisy technique, most people tolerate it well, as it allows better sleep patterns and a subsequent calm demeanor and rested mood.[35]

Thyroid disease

Thyroid disease, hypothyroidism or hyperthyroidism, is a common ailment. In the United States, the prevalence of hypothyroidism is about 3.7% and of hyperthyroidism about 0.5%.[36] Both conditions, more common in women and in the elderly, have broad and systemic effects on the cardiovascular system, cholesterol levels, the metabolic rate, and blood pressure. Approximately 4% of people with hypertension have concomitant hypothyroidism, and the blood pressure in about one-third of these people may normalize with adequate treatment, usually in the form of thyroid hormone replacement.[37] This suggests that about 1% of all people with hypertension have high blood pressure correctible simply by treating their hypothyroidism. In hypertensive people with hypothyroidism, adequate treatment of hypothyroidism may reduce blood pressure by 14/9 mm Hg.[38] However, not all subgroups benefit equally from treatment, as there is a lack of association between hypothyroidism and hypertension in the elderly.[39] This may be due to increased arterial stiffness in elderly people, which itself contributes to elevated blood pressure. An interesting study of people with both hypothyroidism and hypertension supports this view, showing that those with less arterial stiffness had significantly better blood pressure reduction when their hypothyroidism was treated.[40] This suggests that younger people with hypothyroidism may benefit more from treatment. The mechanism of hypothyroid-induced blood pressure elevation is likely from increased sympathetic nervous system activity. Direct stimulation of the adrenal glands to produce aldosterone with subsequent salt and water retention may also contribute.[41]

Considerably less is known about the effects of hyperthyroidism on blood pressure, but a modest increase in systolic blood pressure probably occurs, and some correction may be achieved with restoration of normal thyroid function.[37] Overall, thyroid function should be tested in every person who has hypertension as its treatment alone may correct elevated blood pressure.

Obesity

Obesity has reached epidemic proportions in industrialized societies. Recent data from the National Health and Nutritional Examination Survey (NHANES), which follows health-related trends in the United States, indicate that over 30% of adults in the United States are obese.[42] The risk of hypertension, diabetes, coronary heart disease, and stroke is significantly increased in this population.[43] Overweight and obesity are defined in terms of the body mass index (BMI), which is a measure of a person's weight compared to their height. A BMI of 18.5 to 24.9 kg/m^2 is considered a normal body weight, whereas values from 25 to 29.9 are considered overweight, from 30 to 39.9 as obesity, and anything over 40 as morbid obesity. For example, a man who weighs 80 kg (175 pounds) and is 178 cm (5 feet 10 inches) tall would have a BMI of just over 25 and would be considered overweight. If he weighed 95 kg (210 pounds), his BMI would be over 30 and he would be considered obese. There is a direct and linear progression of blood pressure with BMI.[44] For every 1.7 kg/m^2 increase in men and 1.25 kg/m^2 in women, blood pressure may increase by 1 mm Hg.[45] For example, in the 80 kg (175 pound) and 178 cm (5 feet 10 inches) man previously described, if he gains 5 kg (11 pounds) his blood pressure should increase by 1 mm Hg. The mechanism of obesity-mediated hypertension is complex but is probably caused by activation of the sympathetic nervous system.[46] The RAAS also is activated by sympathetic input to the kidneys and by local production of renin and angiotensin II in adipose tissue.[47] The sum of these actions causes vasoconstriction and retention of salt and water with subsequent blood pressure elevation.

Alcohol

Alcohol has significant cultural and societal importance. Its use is pervasive and its health effects are of great concern. A more complete description of these effects will be discussed in Chapter 8.

Smoking

Smoking is perhaps the most common remediable risk factor for cardiovascular disease and cancer. Over 1 billion people worldwide smoke, with a similar distribution in developing and Western societies. Its association with cardiovascular disease,[48] kidney disease,[49] and cancer are well known, although its effects on blood pressure are less clear. With each cigarette, an immediate rise in blood pressure occurs, peaking within 5 minutes and remaining elevated for up to 15 minutes.[50] The systolic pressure can increase by up to 20 mm Hg.[51] Activation of the sympathetic nervous system by nicotine is regarded as the primary contributing factor.[52] However, the overall effect of smoking on ambulatory blood pressure is less clear, as some studies suggest a lowering of blood pressure,[53] whereas others suggest an increase.[54] This discrepancy may have to do with the age of study subjects, as older smokers tend to have increased blood pressure and younger smokers tend to have lower blood pressure levels.[55] Regardless, the absolute effect is minimal, with a change of only a few millimeters of mercury (mm Hg) in either direction. Surprisingly, former smokers have a higher incidence of hypertension,[56] which may be due to subsequent weight gain following smoking cessation.[57] Despite these seemingly contradictory findings for blood pressure, benefits of smoking cessation in reducing cardiovascular disease and lung cancer are significant.

Caffeine

Caffeine is the most commonly consumed pharmacologically active chemical substance. It is found in beverages such as coffee, tea, sodas, energy drinks, and even some sleep aides. Despite a speculated association with cardiovascular disease, several large studies have concluded that there is no increased risk.[58] In fact, many studies suggest decreased mortality rates in coffee drinkers.[59] The effect of caffeine on the 24-hour ambulatory blood pressure is also debated. Most studies suggest a small increase of up to 2/1 mm Hg in habitual coffee drinkers who drink up to 6 cups a day.[60,61] However, other studies show no increased risk of hypertension.[62] Not disputed is a transient but significant acute increase in blood pressure of up to 10/8 mm Hg,[63] which occurs in occasional coffee or caffeine consumers and in some habitual coffee drinkers after abstaining from caffeine for many hours that occurs with their first morning cup of coffee. People with hypertension and the elderly are more prone to this effect.[64] The mechanism by which caffeine causes such increases is mostly due to activation of the sympathetic nervous system, as mediated by the chemical substance adenosine. Adenosine receptors are found in the brain, the heart, and the blood vessels. When stimulated, they cause deactivation of brain centers, decreased contraction of heart muscle, and relaxation of blood vessels, resulting in a lower blood pressure and a calming effect. It is the agent often given in cardiac stress testing, which causes a compensatory increase in heart rate needed for the study. Caffeine is an adenosine antagonist and blocks the receptors from binding with adenosine, resulting in stimulation of the sympathetic nervous system and constriction of the blood vessels with subsequent blood pressure increase and a more alert state. However, habitual coffee or caffeine users often are tolerant to this effect, as chronic consumption causes a compensatory increase in the number of adenosine receptors.[65] This is likely the reason caffeine has only a mild stimulatory effect and results in only a modest increase in blood pressure in habitual coffee and caffeine consumers.

Nonsteroidal anti-inflammatory drugs

Nonsteroidal anti-inflammatory drugs (NSAIDs) are a complex class of agents. Their primary functions are to treat pain and suppress inflammation. They act by blocking the cyclooxygenase COX-1 and COX-2 enzymes, which are distributed throughout the body in most organs, joints, and muscles. COX-1 mediates clot formation and hemostasis; and COX-2 mediates pain, prevents atherosclerosis, and promotes production of prostaglandins, which collectively dilate blood vessels and promote renal excretion of salt and water resulting in lower blood pressure. NSAIDs inhibit both the COX-1 and COX-2 enzymes, and have different wanted and unwanted effects depending on which enzyme they primarily block. Technically aspirin is an NSAID that primarily blocks the COX-1 enzyme, mostly affecting platelet function and preventing clot formation. By this mechanism it helps prevent heart attack and stroke, although untoward events such as stomach bleeding, stomach ulceration, and brain hemorrhage may occur. Aspirin is not a good analgesic agent as it only minimally blocks the COX-2 enzyme. The more traditional NSAIDs are a group of older drugs that nonselectively block both COX-1 and COX-2 enzymes. Examples include ibuprofen and naproxen, which are common over-the-counter products. They work well in treating pain and inflammation, but also are associated with bleeding and stomach ulcers. A new subgroup of NSAIDs, the COX-2 inhibitors, were designed to address this drawback and primarily (or selectively) block COX-2 enzyme activity. They have good analgesic and anti-inflammatory properties without the unwanted bleeding and stomach ulceration side effects. However, they have been associated with cardiovascular disease, likely due to proatherosclerotic properties from COX-2 inhibition without the compensatory anticlotting effects of COX-1 inhibition.

Although NSAIDs, as a therapeutic class, are commonly recognized for their association with cardiovascular events, worsening of kidney function, and hypertension, the supporting and inculcating data are fragmented and somewhat contradictory, as few clear and nonbiased studies have been conducted. Most clinical trials involve elderly and sick people, with diseases such as rheumatoid arthritis, who may be more prone to adverse effects. Use in younger and healthier people is likely safer. In my practice, I have few concerns recommending this class of medicine to young and healthy people.

Although all NSAIDS are generally associated with cardiovascular disease, several such as ibuprofen and naproxen are relatively safe.[66] The selective COX-2 inhibitors are more strongly associated with cardiovascular events, and rofecoxib (Vioxx) has even been removed from the market.[67] Celecoxib (Celebrex), another commonly used selective COX-2 inhibitor, also has been associated with cardiovascular disease,[68] although other studies refute this claim.[66] The relative safety of celecoxib may arise from it not being strictly a selective COX-2 inhibitor as it partially blocks the COX-1 enzyme as well. However, as this class of medicine shares a large portion of pharmaceutical revenues and is very profitable, many of the studies may be biased in their favor as they are funded by the industry itself. Overall, there likely is an increased risk of cardiovascular disease, especially in people with known cardiovascular risk factors.

NSAIDs are also associated with a decrease in kidney function.[69] Again, some studies with celecoxib report relative safety.[70] In my practice, I discourage any use of NSAIDs in patients with kidney disease.

NSAIDs are associated with modest increases in blood pressure and also block the effects of several classes of blood pressure medications.[71] Again, some studies of celecoxib show no adverse effects.[72] The blood pressure increases, which more commonly occurs in people with kidney disease, and is mostly due to renal salt and water retention.[73] Aldosterone may be an important mediator, as NSAIDs may inhibit its metabolism.[74]

Cocaine abuse

Cocaine is a substrate extracted from the leaves of the erythoxylum coca plant, which is native to South America. Its use by indigenous populations extends back for several centuries. In the mid-19th century, the process of extracting cocaine from its leaf was developed, and thereafter cocaine assumed a role in western society as well. Until the early part of the 20th century, it was added to many beverages, the most famous being coca-cola. It still has medicinal use as an analgesic, although its popularity in this capacity has diminished. Unfortunately, recreational use and abuse has increased in recent years with about 15% of people in the United States having sampled cocaine at some time and about 1% being active users.[75] The health risks most commonly associated with both chronic and acute use of cocaine are cardiovascular. Myocardial ischemia and myocardial infarction are the most frequently noted events, often occurring in young people without prior heart disease. Any young person who suffers a heart attack should be questioned about illicit drug use. Other events include arrhythmia, stroke, dissecting aortic aneurysm, and myocarditis. Cocaine is also associated with kidney disease and is an underestimated cause of kidney failure especially in young people. A sudden and substantial increase in blood pressure and heart rate contributes to these ailments. Depending on the route of administration, its peak effects can occur within a few minutes when inhaled as crack cocaine or when injected intravenously, to about 30 minutes when inhaled nasally. Its primary effect lasts up to 3 hours but its active metabolites peak at a later time and can cause a delayed or second round of events.[76] There are several processes acting to increase blood pressure. In the acute setting, blood norepinephrine levels are increased as its uptake at nerve endings is inhibited. Endothelial dysfunction also contributes to the effect due to suppression of endothelial nitric oxide[77] and increase of endothelin-1 levels.[78] More chronic effects on blood pressure are due to the kidney disease and atherosclerosis that cocaine use can cause.

References

1. Timio M, Saronio P, Venanzi S, Gentili S, Verdura C, Timio F. Blood pressure in nuns in a secluded order: A 30-year follow-up. *Miner Electrolyte Metab.* 1999;25:73–79.
2. Gerin W, Chaplin W, Schwartz JE, et al. Sustained blood pressure increase after an acute stressor: The effects of the 11 September 2001 attack on the New York City World Trade Center. *J Hypertens.* 2005;23:279–284.
3. Cesana G, Sega R, Ferrario M, Chiodini P, Corrao G, Mancia G. Job strain and blood pressure in employed men and women: A pooled analysis of four northern Italian population samples. *Psychosom Med.* 2003;65:558–563.
4. Yan LL, Liu K, Matthews KA, Daviglus ML, Ferguson TF, Kiefe CI. Psychosocial factors and risk of hypertension: The Coronary Artery Risk Development in Young Adults (CARDIA) Study. *JAMA.* 2003;290:2138–2148.
5. Dimsdale JE, Ziegler M, Mills P. Renin correlates with blood pressure reactivity to stressors. *Neuropschopharmacology.* 1990;3:237–242.

6. Schneider MP, Klingbeil AU, Schlaich MP, Langenfeld MR, Veelken R, Schmieder RE. Impaired sodium excretion during mental stress in mild essential hypertension. *Hypertension.* 2001;37:923–927.

7. Ghiadoni L, Donald AE, Cropley M, et al. Mental stress induces transient endothelial dysfunction in humans. *Circulation.* 2000;102:2473–2478.

8. Steptoe A, Marmot M. Impaired cardiovascular recovery following stress predicts 3-year increases in blood pressure. *J Hypertens.* 2005;23:529–536.

9. Palatini P, Palomba D, Bertolo O, et al. The white-coat effect is unrelated to the difference between clinic and daytime blood pressure and is associated with greater reactivity to public speaking. *J Hypertens.* 2003;21:545–553.

10. Mancia G, De Backer G, Dominiczak A, et al. Guidelines for management of arterial hypertension. The Task Force for the Management of Arterial Hypertension of the European Society of Hypertension (ESH) and the European Society of Cardiology (ESC). *Eur Heart J.* 2007;28:1462–1536.

11. Mancia G, Parati G, Pomidossi G, Grassi G, Casadei R, Zanchetti A. Alerting reaction and rise in blood pressure during measurement by physician and nurse. *Hypertension.* 1987;9:209–215.

12. Niiranen TJ, Jula AM, Kantola IM, Reunanen A. Prevalence and determinants of isolated clinic hypertension in the Finnish population: The Finn-HOME study. *J Hypertens.* 2006;24:463–470.

13. Pickering TG, James GD, Boddie C, Harshfield GA, Blank S, Laragh JH. How common is white coat hypertension? *JAMA.* 1988;259:225–228.

14. Verdecchia P, O'Brien E, Pickering T, et al. When can the practicing physician suspect white coat hypertension? Statement from the Working Group on Blood Pressure Monitoring of the European Society of Hypertension. *Am J Hypertens.* 2003;16:87–91.

15. Palatini P, Mormino P, Santonastaso M, et al. Target-organ damage in stage I hypertensive subjects with white coat and sustained hypertension: Results from the HARVEST study. *Hypertension.* 1998;31:57–63.

16. Gustavsen PH, Høegholm A, Bang LE, Kristensen KS. White coat hypertension is a cardiovascular risk factor: A 10-year follow-up study. *J Hum Hypertens.* 2003;17:811–817.

17. Verdecchia P, Reboldi GP, Angeli F, et al. Short- and long-term incidence of stroke in white-coat hypertension. *Hypertension.* 2005;45:203–208.

18. Bidlingmeyer I, Burnier M, Bidlingmeyer M, Waeber B, Brunner HR. Isolated office hypertension: A prehypertensive state? *J Hypertens.* 1996;14:327–332.

19. United Nations, Department of Economic and Social Affairs, Population Division. World contraceptive use. 2007.

20. Mosher WD, Martinez GM, Chandra A, Abma JC, Willson SJ. Use of contraception and use of family planning services in the United States: 1982–2002. *Adv Data.* 2004;350:1–36.

21. WHO Collaborative Study of Cardiovascular Disease and Steroid Hormone Contraception. Acute myocardial infarction and combined oral contraceptives: Results of an international multicentre case-control study. *Lancet.* 1997;349:1202–1209.

22. Gillum LA, Mamidipudi SK, Johnston SC. Ischemic stroke risk with oral contraceptives: A meta-analysis. *JAMA.* 2000;284:72–78.

23. ACOG Committee on Practice Bulletins-Gynecology. Use of hormonal contraception in women with coexisting medical conditions. *Obstet Gynecol.* 2006;107:1453–1472.

24. Ribstein J, Halimi JM, du Cailar G, Mimran A. Renal characteristics and effect of angiotensin suppression in oral contraceptive users. *Hypertension.* 1999;33:90–95.

25. Cardoso F, Polónia J, Santos A, Silva-Carvalho J, Ferreira-de-Almeida J. Low-dose oral contraceptives and 24-hour ambulatory blood pressure. *Int J Gynaecol Obstet.* 1997;59:237–243.

26. Woods JW. Oral contraceptives and hypertension. *Hypertension.* 1998;11(3 Pt 2):II11–15.

27. Young T, Skatrud J, Peppard PE. Risk factors for obstructive sleep apnea in adults. *JAMA.* 2000;291:2013–2016.

28. Peppard PE, Young T, Palta M, Skatrud J. Prospective study of the association between sleep-disordered breathing and hypertension. *N Engl J Med.* 2000;342:1378–1384.

29. Gami AS, Howard DE, Olson EJ, Somers VK. Day-night pattern of sudden death in obstructive sleep apnea. *N Engl J Med.* 2005;352:1206–1214.

30. Somers VK, Dyken ME, Clary MP, Abboud FM. Sympathetic neural mechanisms in obstructive sleep-apnea. *J Clin Invest.* 1995;96:1897–1904.

31. Møller DS, Lind P, Strunge B, Pedersen EB. Abnormal vasoactive hormones and 24-hour blood pressure in obstructive sleep apnea. *Am J Hypertens.* 2003;16:274–280.

32. Calhoun DA, Nishizaka MK, Zaman MA, Harding SM. Aldosterone excretion among subjects with resistant hypertension and symptoms of sleep apnea. *Chest.* 2004;125:112–117.

33. Kato M, Roberts-Thomson P, Phillips BG, et al. Impairment of endothelium-dependent vasodilation of resistance vessels in patients with obstructive sleep apnea. *Circulation.* 2000;102:2607–2610.

34. Pepperell JCT, Ramdassingh-Dow S, Crosthwaite N, et al. Ambulatory blood pressure after therapeutic and subtherapeutic nasal continuous positive airway pressure for obstructive sleep apnoea: A randomized parallel trial. *Lancet.* 2001;359:204–210.

35. Patel SR, White DP, Malhotra A, Stanchina ML, Ayas NT. Continuous positive airway pressure therapy for treating sleepiness in a diverse population with obstructive sleep apnea: Results of a meta-analysis. *Arch Intern Med.* 2003;163:565–571.

36. Aoki Y, Belin RM, Clickner R, Jeffries R, Phillips L, Mahaffey KR. Serum TSH and total T4 in the United States population and their association with participant characteristics: National Health and Nutrition Examination Survey (NHANES 1999–2002). *Thyroid.* 2007;17:1211–1223.

37. Streeten DH, Anderson GH Jr, Howland T, Chiang R, Smulyan H. Effects of thyroid function on blood pressure: Recognition of hypothyroid hypertension. *Hypertension.* 1988;11:78–83.

38. Saito I, Ito K, Saruta T. Hypothyroidism as a cause of hypertension. *Hypertension.* 1983;5:112–115.

39. Bergus GR, Mold JW, Barton ED, Randall CS. The lack of association between hypertension and hypothyroidism in a primary care setting. *J Hum Hypertens.* 1999;13:231–235.

40. Dernellis J, Panaretou M. Effects of thyroid replacement therapy on arterial blood pressure in patients with hypertension and hypothyroidism. *Am Heart J.* 2002;143:718–724.

41. Fommei E, Iervasi G. The role of thyroid hormone in blood pressure homeo-stasis: Evidence from short-term hypothyroidism in humans. *J Clin Endocrinol Metab*. 2002;87:1996–2000.

42. Flegal KM, Carroll MD, Ogden CL, Curtin LR. Prevalence and trends in obe-sity among U.S. adults, 1999–2008. *JAMA*. 2010;303:235–241.

43. Thompson D, Edelsberg J, Colditz GA, Bird AP, Oster G. Lifetime health and economic consequences of obesity. *Arch Intern Med*. 1999;159:2177–2183.

44. Bays HE, Chapman RH, Grandy S, SHIELD Investigators' Group. The rela-tionship of body mass index to diabetes mellitus, hypertension and dys-lipidaemia: Comparison of data from two national surveys. *Int J Clin Pract*. 2007;61:737–747.

45. Doll S, Paccaud F, Bovet P, Burnier M, Wietlisbach V. Body mass index, abdominal adiposity and blood pressure: Consistency of their association across developing countries. *Int J Obesity*. 2002;26:48–57.

46. Rahmouni K, Correia ML, Haynes WG, Mark AL. Obesity-associated hyper-tensions: New insights into mechanisms. *Hypertension*. 2005;45:9–14.

47. Engeli S, Negrel R, Sharma AM. Physiology and patophysiology of the adi-pose tissue renin-angiotensin system. *Hypertension*. 2000;35:1270–1277.

48. Teo KK, Ounpuu S, Hawken S, et al. Tobacco use and risk of myocardial infarction in 52 countries in the INTERHEART study: A case-control study. *Lancet*. 2006;368:647–658.

49. Orth SR, Ritz E. The renal risks of smoking: An update. *Curr Opion Nephrol Hypertens*. 2002;11:483–488.

50. Mahmud A, Feely J. Effects of smoking on arterial stiffness and pulse pres-sure amplification. *Hypertension*. 2003;41:183–187.

51. Groppelli A, Giorgi DM, Omboni S, Parati G, Mancia G. Persistent blood pressure increase induced by heavy smoking. *J Hypertens*. 1992;10:495–499.

52. Najem B, Houssiere A, Pathak A, et al. Acute cardiovascular and sympathetic effects of nicotine replacement therapy. *Hypertension*. 2006;47:1162–1167.

53. Green MS, Jucha E, Luz Y. Blood pressure in smokers and nonsmokers: Epidemiologic findings. *Am Heart J*. 1986;111:932–940.

54. Verdecchia P, Schillaci G, Borgioni C, et al. Cigarette smoking, ambula-tory blood pressure and cardiac hypertrophy in essential hypertension. *J Hyperten*. 1995;13:1209–1216.

55. Primatesta P, Falaschetti E, Gupta S, Marmot MG, Poulter NR. Association between smoking and blood pressure: Evidence from the health survey for England. *Hypertension*. 2001;37:187–193.

56. Lee DH, Ha MH, Kim JR, Jacobs DR Jr. Effects of smoking cessation on changes in blood pressure and incidence of hypertension: A 4-year follow-up study. *Hypertension*. 2001;37:194–198.

57. Halimi JM, Giraudeau B, Vol S, Cacès E, Nivet H, Tichet J. The risk of hyper-tension in men: Direct and indirect effects of chronic smoking. *J Hypertens*. 2002;20:187–193.

58. Lopez-Garcia E, van Dam RM, Willett WC, et al. Coffee consumption and coronary heart disease in men and women: A prospective cohort study. *Circulation*. 2006;113:2045–2053.

59. Lopez-Garcia E, van Dam RM, Li TY, Rodriguez-Artalejo F, Hu FB. The relationship of coffee consumption with mortality. *Ann Intern Med*. 2008;148:904–914.

60. Noordzij M, Uiterwaal CS, Arends LR, Kok FJ, Grobbee DE, Geleijnse JM. Blood pressure response to chronic intake of coffee and caffeine: A meta-analysis of randomized controlled trials. *J Hypertens.* 2005;23:921–928.
61. van Dusseldorp M, Smits P, Thien T, Katan MB. Effect of decaffeinated versus regular coffee on blood pressure: A 12-week, double-blind trial. *Hypertension.* 1989;14:563–569.
62. Winkelmayer WC, Stampfer MJ, Willett WC, Curhan GC. Habitual caffeine intake and the risk of hypertension in women. *JAMA.* 2005;294:2330–2335.
63. Hartley TR, Sung BH, Pincomb GA, Whitsett TL, Wilson MF, Lovallo WR. Hypertension risk status and effect of caffeine on blood pressure. *Hypertension.* 2000;36:137–141.
64. Rakic V, Burke V, Beilin LJ. Effects of coffee on ambulatory blood pressure in older men and women: A randomized controlled trial. *Hypertension.* 1999;33:869–873.
65. Ammon HP. Biochemical mechanism of caffeine tolerance. *Arch Pharm (Weinheim).* 1991;324:261–267.
66. McGettigan P, Henry D. Cardiovascular risk and inhibition of cyclooxygenase: A systemic review of the observational studies of selective and nonselective inhibitors of cyclooxygenase 2. *JAMA.* 2006;29:1633–1644.
67. Bresalier RS, Sandler RS, Quan H, et al. Cardiovascular events associated with Rofecoxib in a colorectal adenoma chemoprevention trial. *N Engl J Med.* 2005;352:1092–1102.
68. Solomon SD, McMurray JJ, Pfeffer MA, et al. Cardiovascular risk associated with Celecoxib in a clinical trial for colorectal adenoma prevention. *N Engl J Med.* 2005; 352:1071–1080.
69. Schwartz JI, Vandormael K, Malice MP, et al. Comparison of rofecoxib, celecoxib and naproxen on renal function in elderly subjects receiving a normal-salt diet. *Clin Pharmacol Ther.* 2002;72:50–61.
70. Whelton A, Schulman G, Wallemark C, et al. Effects of Celecoxib and Naproxen on renal function in the elderly. *Arch Intern Med.* 2000;160:1465–1470.
71. Johnson AG, Nguyen TV, Day RO. Do nonsteroidal anti-inflammatory drugs affect blood pressure? A meta-analysis. *Ann Intern Med.* 1994;121:289–300.
72. Sowers JR, White WB, Pitt B, et al. The effects of cyclooxygenase-2 inhibitors and nonsteroidal anti-inflammatory therapy on 24-hour blood pressure in patients with hypertension, osteoarthritis, and type 2 diabetes mellitus. *Arch Intern Med.* 2005;165:161–168.
73. White WB. Cardiovascular effects of the cyclooxygenase inhibitors. *Hypertension.* 2007;49:408–418.
74. Knights KM, Mangoni AA, Miners JO. Non-selective nonsteroidal anti-inflammatory drugs and cardiovascular events: Is aldosterone the silent partner in crime? *Br J Clin Pharmacol.* 2006;61:738–740.
75. Jaffe JA, Kimmel PL. Chronic nephropathies of cocaine and heroin abuse: A critical review. *Clin J Am Soc Nephrol.* 2006;1:655–667.
76. Lange RA, Hillis D. Cardiovascular complications of cocaine use. *N Engl J Med.* 2001;345:351–358.
77. Mo W, Singh AK, Arruda JA, Dunea G. Role of nitric oxide in cocaine-induced acute hypertension. *Am J Hypertens.* 1998;11(6 Pt 1):708–714.

78. Wilbert-Lampen U, Seliger C, Zilker T, Arendt RM. Cocaine increases the endothelial release of immunoreactive endothelin and its concentrations in human plasma and urine: Reversal by coincubation with sigma-receptor antagonists. *Circulation.* 1998;98:385–390.

chapter four

Blood pressure medications

Modern medicine offers several classes of blood pressure medications. As described in Chapter 2, Poiseuille's law characterizes blood pressure in terms of the volume of blood transported in the vessels (i.e., the cardiac output [CO]) and the resistance (or degree of constriction) of the vessels. Either factor can independently affect the blood pressure. For example, a high salt and water intake in a salt-sensitive person raises the blood pressure by increasing the blood volume. In most people, hypertension is due to a combination of both factors, although one often predominates. Of note, the epidemic of hypertension is a relatively recent occurrence, as just a few centuries ago only a small percentage of people suffered from it. In fact, humans historically had very low blood pressure requiring them to consume salt and fluid to maintain an adequate blood pressure. Imagine our ancestors who lived in hot arid climates without free-flowing water or an adequate food supply. They were dehydrated most of the time. Therefore, our genomic structure is modeled around mechanisms that retain salt and raise blood pressure. It is only in recent times that salt has been consumed in excess and that people are living to older ages that we are suffering from this widespread prevalence of hypertension. The two factors of Poiseuille's law can be viewed as a defense mechanism to prevent low blood pressure. Laragh and his colleagues have eloquently developed the mechanisms of hypertension and methods to approach its treatment.[1] They classify each type of blood pressure medication into two groups depending on the component of blood pressure they primarily affect.[2,3] Medicines that decrease the resistance (or degree of constriction) of the blood vessel are referred to as R (or renin) type, as the renin–angiotensin system (RAS) primarily acts to sustain blood pressure by constricting the blood vessels. Blocking this system causes reduced vascular resistance and lowered blood pressure. Examples of R-type medicine classes include angiotensin-converting enzyme (ACE) inhibitors, angiotensin II receptor blockers (ARBs), direct renin inhibitors (DRIs), and beta blockers, which all block a part of the renin–angiotensin pathway. V-type medicines comprise all other non-R-type medicines and include diuretics and several classes that are primarily vasodilators. Laragh proposes using plasma levels of the enzyme renin as a guide to classifying the etiology of hypertension and in choosing appropriate treatment. However, as normal plasma renin levels are quite low, accurate measurement of its levels are difficult. Previous attempts to do

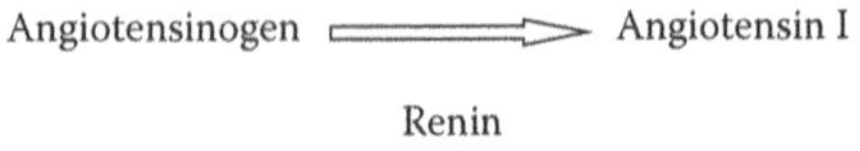

Angiotensinogen ⇌ Angiotensin I

Renin

Figure 4.1 Renin-mediated conversion of angiotensinogen to angiotensin.

so have led to inaccuracies, and may have led to confusion as to its role in regulating blood pressure and mediating hypertension. Laragh and his colleagues, therefore, helped pioneer the plasma renin activity (PRA), which is an assay that estimates the activity of plasma renin by measuring the hourly conversion of angiotensinogen to angiotensin I (Figure 4.1). The PRA is currently considered the gold standard for estimating renin levels and also can be used to characterize the etiology of hypertension. An elevated PRA suggests an RAS-mediated etiology and an R-type medicine should be initiated in treatment, whereas a low PRA suggests a non-RAS (i.e., salt or volume mediated) etiology, suggesting selection of a V-type medicine. Use of the PRA provides a methodical and scientific approach to treating hypertension. Unfortunately, many physicians randomly add medicines without a logical rationale or an adequate response. Laragh's method provides a rational approach to treating hypertension and should lead to the use of fewer medicines.

The various classes of blood pressure medications currently used all have been well characterized with the rigors and expenses of scientific research. Their efficacy and side effects are well characterized. These therapies sometimes offer unique benefit and protection for specific diseases. For example, several offer better protection from cardiac disease, whereas others help protect against stroke or kidney disease. Despite this variation, there is considerable evidence that the absolute reduction in blood pressure itself is more important in reducing overall cardiovascular disease than the specific class of medicine used.[4] Natural or holistic medicines and techniques are usually based on time-honored experience and response, but the rigors of science are often not available to define them. Therefore, they have often been relegated as nonscientific. With classification of these modalities in terms of R or V types, they may be viewed in a more scientific way. This chapter will classify the types of modern medicines in this way and their respective mechanisms of action and side effect profiles will be described. The following chapters will then characterize alternative medicines and techniques according to the same parameters, thus adding a measure of scientific validity to their use.

Diuretics

Diuretics are the most commonly used class of blood pressure medication. Their popularity is due to time-proven effectiveness and relatively modest cost. They lower blood pressure by promoting salt and water excretion

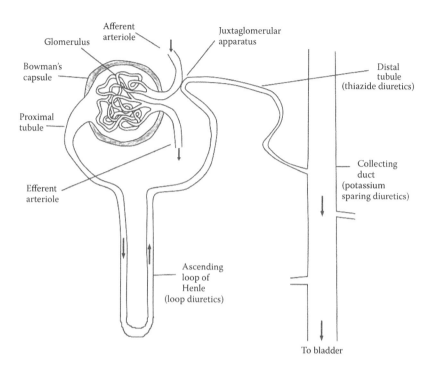

Figure 4.2 Schematic of the nephron. (Courtesy of Shani Strenger from Shilo, Israel.)

by the kidneys and are considered V-type medicines. However, their use is limited by their side effects that mostly occur at higher dosages. As described in Chapter 2, each kidney is composed of about 1 million nephrons, each of which processes a small fraction of the plasma filtrate and collectively contributes to the daily urine pool. The nephron is made of the glomerulus, which filters the blood and the tubule, which then reabsorbs needed nutrients such as electrolytes and water, and leaves toxins and waste products to be eliminated (Figure 4.2).

In an average healthy man the kidneys filter about 180 liters (50 gallons) of plasma and about 600 grams (1.3 pounds) of sodium per day. This amounts to far more fluid and sodium than is present in the entire body and without subsequent processing by the tubules to reclaim these elements, we would quickly dehydrate. Diuretics work by blocking this reabsorption process, causing increased sodium and water excretion. There are three basic types of diuretics, each affecting a different segment of the tubule—thiazides, loop diuretics, and potassium-sparing diuretics (Table 4.1). Thiazides are the most popular type of diuretic as they provide a prolonged, steady, and gentle lowering of blood pressure. They block reabsorption at the distal convoluted tubule segment. Loop diuretics are

Table 4.1 Diuretics

Thiazide diuretics	Loop diuretics	Potassium sparing diuretics
Hydroclorothiazide	Furosemide	Spironolactone
Chlorothiazide	Torsemide	Eplerenone
Metolazone	Bumetanide	Amiloride
Indapamide	Ethacrynic acid	Triamterene

also popular and are very potent diuretics that promote large and rapid excretion of electrolytes and water. They act at an earlier segment of the tubule called the ascending loop of Henle. Potassium-sparing diuretics have recently regained acceptance and popularity. They minimize potassium losses by blocking the collecting ducts in the final tubule segment. Their action is the slowest, often taking several months to reach peak effect. Combinations of diuretics can be used for a more robust response.

A typical response to diuretic use in a person with hypertension is a lowering of systolic/diastolic blood pressure by about 15/10 mm Hg, although there is variability between different races.[5] Diuretics have been proven efficacious in preventing the onset of cardiovascular disease in people with hypertension[6] and are the preferred class of blood pressure medication in well-regarded studies.[7] Hypokalemia, which arises from urinary loss of potassium, is the most common side effect for all but the potassium-sparing diuretics, and many caregivers prescribe a potassium supplement *de novo* when initiating diuretic therapy. This used to be more common when higher diuretic doses were prescribed. Arrhythmias, sudden cardiac death,[8] and stroke[9] occur more commonly in people with hypokalemia. Another side effect is a possible increase in blood glucose levels,[10] although there is no overt increased risk of developing diabetes itself when low to moderate doses are used.[11] Cholesterol levels may also become elevated.[12] A particularly vexing problem associated with many blood pressure medicines is sexual dysfunction, especially in men. Of all types of blood pressure medication, only diuretics may have a legitimate association with erectile dysfunction,[13] although the effect is relatively short in duration lasting up to 2 years. Gout is also more common with diuretic use.[14] Other electrolytes such as sodium[15] and magnesium[16] may become depleted with diuretic use so their levels need to be monitored during therapy with these agents.

Calcium channel blockers

The calcium channel blockers have been used to treat hypertension since the 1980s. They have relatively few side effects, making them a well-tolerated and popular class of medicine. They work by blocking the movement of calcium into the smooth muscle cells of the arterial blood vessels

Table 4.2 Calcium Channel Blockers

Dihydropyridines	Nondihydropyridines
Amlodipine	Diltiazem
Felodipine	Verapamil
Nifedipine	

and the myocardium through channels embedded in the cell membranes that regulate the flux of calcium into the cells. Intracellular calcium levels affect the contractility of muscle cells, with higher levels causing more contraction. In the smooth muscle cells of the blood vessels, calcium influx regulates the diameter of the vessels and consequently their resistance. Similarly, calcium determines the force and rate of the contraction of myocardial cells and consequently alters the CO. There are two subtypes of calcium channel blockers, the dihydropyridines and the nondihydropyridines, which differ by binding to different parts of the channel. The dihydropyridines more selectively target blood vessels and therefore act as vasodilators, whereas the nondihydropyridines primarily affect the cardiac muscle and therefore reduce contractility, heart rate, and CO. They are potent antihypertensive medicines and can lower the systolic/diastolic blood pressure by 14–15/10–13 mm Hg.[5] Calcium channel blockers are V-type medications as they lower blood pressure without blocking the RAS and may even have some diuretic properties (see Table 4.2).

Older studies suggest that use of these drugs may be associated with increased rates of myocardial infarction[17] and mortality.[18,19] However, in fairness to this therapeutic class, these studies were done using the older and shorter-acting formulations. Blood levels of these drugs would quickly increase and decrease, causing large swings in blood pressure, which likely contributed to the reported adverse events. These short-acting medications are no longer commonly used. Several more recent, respected studies using the newer and longer-acting versions, such as amlodipine, show similar cardiovascular protection in people with hypertension when compared with other classes of medication.[7] In fact, some studies even suggest that amlodipine provides better cardiovascular protection than ACE inhibitors.[20] Calcium channel blockers also help in regressing cardiac hypertrophy,[21] are particularly useful in preventing stroke in people with hypertension,[22] and may protect against the onset of dementia.[23] A common side effect is swelling, which occurs predominantly in the lower extremities.[24] Some studies suggest an association with developing cancers[25] and gastrointestinal bleeding,[26] but these claims are widely disputed. Despite a direct cause and effect between hypertension and kidney disease, the calcium channel blockers, although effective in lowering blood pressure, do not protect from kidney disease as well as other classes of antihypertensive medications.[27] This is probably due to

Table 4.3 Alpha Blockers

| Doxazosin |
| Prazosin |
| Terazosin |

preferential dilation of the small arterioles that lead into the kidneys causing elevated pressure within the glomerulus. This condition, known as hyperfiltration, causes increased stress and kidney scarring.[28]

Alpha blockers

The alpha blockers are a class of blood pressure medication often used as a secondary option and only rarely as the primary choice (see Table 4.3). They act by blocking the alpha-1 receptors of the smooth muscle cells of the blood vessels. These receptors are activated by norepinephrine, systemically produced by the adrenal glands and locally by nerve cell endings adjacent to the vessel walls. When the body is physically or emotionally stressed, norepinephrine levels increase through stimulation of the sympathetic nervous system. Activating the alpha-1 receptors cause the smooth muscle cells to contract, which in turn causes vasoconstriction and subsequent blood pressure elevation (Figure 4.3).

The alpha blockers disrupt this process, causing vasodilation and blood pressure lowering. A typical response can lower the systolic/diastolic blood pressure by 15/12 mmHg.[5] Alpha blockers are V-type medicines. Prior to 2000, the alpha blockers were a common choice. However, a well-publicized preliminary report from the influential ALLHAT Collaborative Research Group suggested that doxazosin, an alpha blocker, was associated with increased risk of developing cardiovascular events, particularly congestive heart failure.[29] Although this outcome is still debated, the alpha blockers have since been relegated to a secondary role in treating hypertension.[30] However, they have been used effectively as adjunctive treatment for people with blood pressure inadequately controlled by other standard therapy.[31] Despite the bad press given to this class, it does have unique properties that make it attractive. Alpha blockers significantly lower cholesterol levels[32] and have favorable effects on

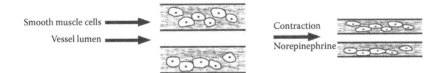

Figure 4.3 Regulation of arteriole lumen diameter by smooth muscle cells, mediated by norepinephrine. (Courtesy of Shani Strenger from Shilo, Israel.)

diabetes and insulin sensitivity,[33] two parameters that are often worsened by other blood pressure medications. They also benefit men with enlarged hypertrophic prostates, as they relax the prostate muscle and reduce symptoms of urinary frequency. In fact, several alpha blockers are marketed solely for the treatment of this condition. Of all the classes of blood pressure medication, they are least associated with sexual dysfunction and may even benefit men with erectile problems.[13] Untoward side effects include postural hypotension[34] and urinary incontinence in women.[35] The former can be a vexing problem, especially in the elderly, and I try to avoid its use in this population.

Direct vasodilators

The direct vasodilators are an eclectic class of antihypertensive medication comprised of several relatively unrelated medicines that have been in use for decades. The most common ones are hydralazine, minoxidil, and the nitrates. They are V-type medicines that lower blood pressure by dilating the blood vessels, each drug with its own distinct mechanism of action. This effect is often brisk and large, causing a compensatory response with activation of the sympathetic nervous system and the RAS. The resulting increased heart contractility, heart rate, and fluid retention cause a compensatory rise in blood pressure, negating some of the intended effect and potentially adding strain on the heart as well. Therefore, they are not used as primary agents for lowering blood pressure and instead are used adjunctively with diuretics or other medications that suppress the sympathetic nervous system, such as beta blockers.

Hydralazine and the nitrates both dilate the vessels by increasing nitric oxide levels within the smooth muscle cells. Hydralazine works indirectly by inhibiting production of substances such as reactive oxygen species, which themselves degrade nitric oxide. It has found a niche in treating pregnant women as it is relatively safe to fetal development. It also is commonly used in intravenous form to rapidly lower blood pressure in emergent states of hypertension. An important side effect, which significantly restricts its use, is occurrence of lupus-like symptoms.[36] This occurs more commonly in women and with use of high doses, only rarely occurring with low doses. As these symptoms infrequently occur before 6 months, low doses of hydralazine can be safely used in most pregnancies. Fortunately, these symptoms fully resolve when the medicine is stopped. The nitrates dilate blood vessels by directly releasing nitric oxide molecules, which are embedded in their chemical structure, into the smooth muscle cells. They are primarily used in treating angina symptoms in people with heart disease, despite an ability to potently reduce blood pressure. Perhaps the most serious drawback to their use is the development of tolerance when prescribed continuously throughout the day.[37]

This significantly decreases their effectiveness in lowering blood pressure as the body becomes inured to elevated levels of nitric oxide. Their use, therefore, is limited to relatively short-acting forms of drugs and is dosed so that their effect lasts only a part of the day. This clearly makes them unappealing in treating hypertension. An important study of black people with heart failure showed a significant benefit in adding hydralazine to nitrate use.[38] Mortality rates in these very sick people were reduced by nearly half. It is speculated that hydralazine, through its ability to protect from nitric oxide degradation, diminishes the effects of nitrate tolerance resulting in improved health outcomes.[39] A combination pill of hydralazine and isosorbide dinitrate is available, although it is far more expensive than the individual formulations.

Minoxidil is perhaps the most potent antihypertensive agent and its use is usually reserved for treating very difficult-to-control hypertension.[40] Similar to other vasodilators, it causes an increased heart rate as well as salt and fluid retention, and therefore should be accompanied by a diuretic or a beta blocker. An interesting side effect is hair growth, which has led to topical minoxidil becoming a popular treatment for baldness. Unfortunately, it is associated with the development of pericardial effusion, which can be a serious problem.

Renin–angiotensin system blockade

The following sections describe four related classes of blood pressure medicines that block the RAS, including ACE inhibitors, ARBs, DRIs, and beta blockers. As described in Chapter 2, the RAS is a complex system involving several enzymes, substrates, and chemical messengers (Figure 4.4). Its primary function in controlling blood pressure is to regulate arteriolar resistance, although it secondarily affects aldosterone production and consequently fluid balance. All four classes are R-type medications, although each blocks the RAS at different points. Plasma renin levels control the

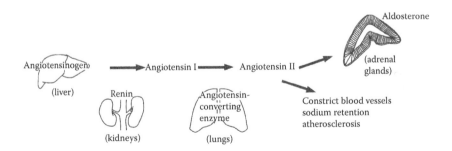

Figure 4.4 The renin–angiotensin(–aldosterone) system. (Courtesy of Shani Strenger from Shilo, Israel.)

throughput of this system as this part of the process is the rate-limiting step for the entire system. As previously noted, the PRA is the current gold standard laboratory test that estimates the renin levels.

Angiotensin-converting enzyme (ACE) inhibitors

ACE inhibitors block the RAS by inhibiting the function of the angiotensin-converting enzyme, thereby preventing the conversion of angiotensin I to angiotensin II (Figure 4.5). Paradoxically, these agents cause an increase in the PRA, as decreased levels of angiotensin II blunt its usual negative feedback on renin production. They can lower systolic/diastolic blood pressure in people with hypertension by 13/10 mm Hg, although somewhat less in black people.[5] This class of drugs has particular protective effects from kidney disease[41] and reduces the rate of decline in kidney function in people with diabetic[42] and nondiabetic[43] nephropathy. ACE inhibitors also have unique cardiovascular protective effects and benefit people who have suffered from a heart attack[44] or who have congestive heart failure.[45] Overall, it is a well-tolerated class with few side effects and its quality-of-life measures superior to most other classes.[46] Two common and serious side effects, occurring mostly in people with kidney disease, are elevated blood potassium levels and worsening of kidney function.[47] Both effects are reversible but can be serious and often lead to discontinuation of the medicine. Perhaps the most serious side effect is angioedema, which is a sudden onset of generalized swelling. It can occlude the breathing airways and rapidly cause suffocation and death if not treated promptly. Fortunately, it only occurs in about 1 in 1000 people taking ACE inhibitors,[48] although it is more common in black people.[49] A dry cough is a more common side effect and occurs in up to 5% to 20% of people.[50] Chinese people are most prone to this effect, which occurs in up to half of those taking ACE inhibitors.[51] In addition, this class of drugs should not be used in pregnant women as they are associated with fetal

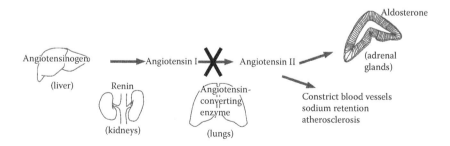

Figure 4.5 Angiotensin-converting enzyme inhibition. (Courtesy of Shani Strenger from Shilo, Israel.)

Table 4.4 Angiotensin-Converting Enzyme Inhibitors

Captopril
Enalapril
Benazepril
Fosinopril
Lisinopril
Ramipril
Trandolapril
Quinapril

complications.[52] In my practice, I try to avoid their use in women of child-bearing age. ACE inhibitors cause decreased red blood cell production and may lead to anemia.[53] They are associated with low glucose levels in people with diabetes,[54] which should be monitored carefully. Compared with most other classes they may be protective of developing diabetes (see Table 4.4).[55]

Angiotensin II receptor blockers (ARBs)

ARBs (Table 4.5) block the RAS by inhibiting the binding of angiotensin II to its receptor (Figure 4.6). This lowers blood pressure by preventing vaso-constriction. Like the ACE inhibitors, they too paradoxically increase the PRA. They share many properties with the ACE inhibitors, both beneficial and harmful, and they lower blood pressure by a comparable amount. However, there are several differences that set the two classes apart. Like ACE inhibitors, ARBs are well tolerated and provide a superior quality-of-life measure compared with other classes. They have the lowest attrition rate of all classes of blood pressure medications[56] and provide significant protective effects from kidney disease, especially in patients with diabetes with advanced kidney disease.[57] Surprisingly, a few studies suggest poor cardiovascular protection and some even suggest an increased risk of adverse events. However, most studies show superior cardiovascular benefit and suggest preventive effects from the onset of cardiovascular disease.[58] Due to this discrepancy many physicians, especially cardiologists, prefer to use ACE inhibitors but will consider an ARB as a second

Table 4.5 Angiotensin II Receptor Blockers

Candesartan
Irbesartan
Losartan
Olmesartan
Telmisartan
Valsartan

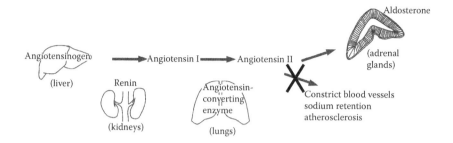

Figure 4.6 Angiotensin II receptor blockade. (Courtesy of Shani Strenger from Shilo, Israel.)

choice in people with advanced cardiovascular disease.[59] Most ARBs have a relatively short half-life, and despite being marketed for once-daily use, their blood levels drop rapidly and usually do not last a full 24 hours. As heart attacks occur most commonly in the morning hours between 6 A.M. and noon, it may be that inadequate levels of ARBs during this crucial period contribute to their diminished cardiovascular protecting ability. I often suggest to my patients who use the shorter-acting ARBs to divide the dose and take twice daily. Reversible kidney dysfunction and elevated blood potassium levels occur but to a lesser degree than with ACE inhibitors.[60] Angioedema and cough also occur,[61] but much less so than with ACE inhibitors. Maternal exposure should be limited, as ARBs also have fetal toxic effects.[62] Beneficial effects in patients with diabetes also exist.[63]

Direct renin inhibitors (DRIs)

The DRIs are a relatively new and exciting class of blood pressure medication. They block the RAS by directly inhibiting the function of the enzyme renin (Figure 4.7). By disrupting the system at an early stage, they limit production of angiotensin II altogether and also lower the PRA. Aliskiren (Tekturna) is an example of a DRI that has received FDA approval. Its

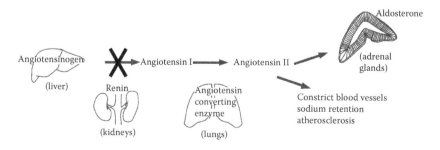

Figure 4.7 Direct renin inhibition. (Courtesy of Shani Strenger from Shilo, Israel.)

ability to lower blood pressure is comparable to ACE inhibitors and ARBs, with reduction in systolic/diastolic blood pressure of 15/11 mm Hg.[64] As it is relatively new, studies are still being conducted but the anticipated kidney and cardiovascular protective effects are presumed comparable to those of the ACE inhibitors and ARBs. There is evidence of protection from kidney disease progression in people with diabetes[65] and for cardiovascular benefit.[66] Aliskiren is well tolerated and has few side effects. Diarrhea, headache, and dizziness may occur but are relatively uncommon.[67] Similar to ACE inhibitors and ARBs, there is some risk of reversible kidney dysfunction and elevated potassium levels. Aliskiren has a very long half-life, so adequate coverage over an entire 24-hour period should enable once-daily dosing.

Beta blockers

Along with diuretics, beta blockers are one of the blood pressure medications in use since the 1960s. It is a complex class, comprised of many agents that each has unique properties. It is difficult to categorize them uniformly because the benefits and side-effect profiles differ within the class. These agents work by blocking the beta-1 receptors, which are found in the kidneys, heart, and brain. Circulating norepinephrine (and epinephrine), produced by the nervous system and the adrenal glands, activate these receptors and cause increased renin production by the kidneys, more rapid and stronger contraction of the heart, and enhanced stimulation of the brain centers, with a cumulative effect of increasing blood pressure. By blocking these receptors, the beta blockers cause decreased renin production by the kidneys, a slower heart rate, and diminished heart contraction, which together decrease plasma renin levels and the CO. These effects contribute to a lowered blood pressure and decreased strain on the heart. Despite having a combined R- and V-type effect in lowering blood pressure, they are classified as R-type medicines as renin levels are reduced. They can lower systolic/diastolic blood pressure in people with hypertension by 15/12 mm Hg.[5] Unfortunately, many of these agents are not specific in blocking the beta-1 receptors and often also block the beta-2 receptors, which cause unwanted side effects. The newer beta blockers are far more specific to the beta-1 receptor and some even have other favorable blood-pressure-lowering properties (see Table 4.6).

Because this therapeutic class is not as homogeneous as others, there is confusion and debate about its role in treating hypertension. Many think the beta blockers should not be used in treating primary (uncomplicated) hypertension, as some studies show no protective effect from the onset of cardiovascular disease or stroke.[68] However, most of these studies used one particular beta blocker, atenolol, which for several reasons is not ideal and perhaps misrepresents the class.[69] Most other beta

Table 4.6 Beta Blockers

Atenolol
Bisoprolol
Carvedilol
Labetalol
Metoprolol (Toprol)
Propanolol

blockers, especially the newer ones, show significant benefit in protection against the onset of cardiovascular disease. Yet, despite this ambiguity, they clearly are protective in people with existing cardiovascular disease, regardless of whether they have normal or elevated blood pressure. They are the agent of choice for people who have had a heart attack[70] or who have congestive heart failure.[71] By slowing the heart rate and by reducing the contractile forces of the heart, they reduce the overall cardiac stress and workload, and decrease the occurrence of abnormal and often lethal arrhythmias. In people undergoing surgery who have risk factors for heart disease, beta blockers also decrease the likelihood of perioperative heart attacks.[72] Unfortunately, they are associated with many untoward side effects and are often not well tolerated. Abrupt withdrawal of beta blockers can cause a rebound effect resulting in sudden blood pressure elevation and tachycardia, which can cause angina symptoms and even a heart attack.[73] Historically, beta blockers are associated with respiratory problems, especially in people with asthma or emphysema. However, the newer more selective ones are much safer and usually well tolerated even in people with lung disease.[74] Perhaps the most serious problem is their association with elevated glucose levels and diabetes.[75] Beta blockers also may cause elevated cholesterol levels, particularly the triglycerides.[76] These two serious side effects may be the reason that this class poorly prevents the onset of cardiovascular disease, as the benefits of lowering blood pressure and reducing heart strain may be compromised by higher glucose and cholesterol levels. Last, beta blockers are associated with decreased exercise endurance and a generalized feeling of fatigue.[77] Overall, it is a very complicated class of blood pressure medication, and although associated with many problems, beta blockers are useful if chosen wisely.

Central alpha agonists

The central alpha agonists are another older class of blood pressure medication in use for many decades. They were commonly used in the 1960s and 1970s but mostly have been replaced by newer classes due to intolerable side effects. Clonidine and methyldopa are the two more common

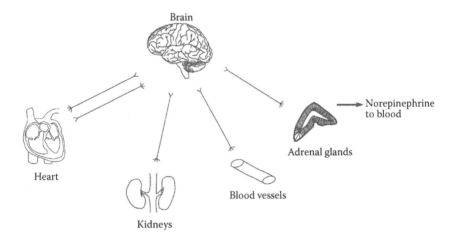

Figure 4.8 Regulation of body organ function by the sympathetic nervous system. (Courtesy of Shani Strenger from Shilo, Israel.)

agents within this class and still are used. They lower blood pressure by blocking the sympathetic output of the central nervous system, and their efficacy is comparable to most other classes. As previously described, several brain centers regulate the output of the sympathetic nervous system to various organs. When stimulated, the terminal nerve endings release norepinephrine and activate the alpha-1 and beta-1 receptors of the blood vessels, kidneys, heart, and adrenal glands causing blood pressure elevation (Figure 4.8).

The central alpha agonists block this process early in its action pathway. The drugs pass the blood–brain barrier and activate the alpha-2 receptors of the regulating brain centers, thereby turning off the sympathetic nervous system outflow. Similar to the beta blockers, they cause decreased production of renin by the kidneys, a slower heart rate, and diminished heart contraction, which together decrease plasma renin levels and the CO. Despite having a combined R- and V-type effect in lowering blood pressure, they are classified as R-type medicines as renin levels are reduced. A common side effect of these agents is drowsiness and sedation, which many find difficult to tolerate. Dry mouth, depression, and sexual impotence also occur relatively frequently. Therefore, central alpha agonists mostly have been replaced with the newer and more palatable classes of medicines. Other side effects include bradycardia[78] and hepatitis, particularly with methyldopa.[79] A rebound effect may occur if the medicines are abruptly stopped, and the blood pressure and heart rate may exceed levels prior to starting them.[80] Consequently, it is important to slowly reduce the dosage when electing to stop these medicines to avoid these negative effects. Despite this, the central alpha blockers have many favorable properties and have found a unique niche. Clonidine rapidly and efficiently lowers blood pressure, and is often used as an alternative to intravenous blood pressure medications in treating urgent and emergent hypertension.[81] Given its sedating properties, clonidine also has utility in treating symptoms arising from withdrawal from alcohol, tobacco, and opiate drugs.[82] It also may reduce hot flashes in women with breast cancer receiving hormone therapy.[83] Methyldopa has maintained a niche in treating pregnant women with hypertension, as it is relatively safe to the fetus.

A relatively new class of centrally acting medicines is the imidazoline receptor agonists. The imidazoline receptors also are found in brain centers that regulate the sympathetic nervous system. Their function is similar to alpha-2 receptors but activation of these receptors causes significantly fewer side effects. Unfortunately, these drugs are not available in many countries, including the United States, in large part due to a study of people with existent heart failure in which a significant number died while taking the medication.[84]

References

1. Laragh J. Laragh's lessons in pathophysiology and clinical pearls for treating hypertension. *Am J Hypertens*. 2001;14:84–89.
2. Laragh JH, Sealey JE. The plasma renin test reveals the contribution of body sodium-volume content (V) and renin–angiotensin (R) vasoconstriction to long-term blood pressure. *Am J Hypertens*. 2011;24:1164–1180.
3. Laragh J. Laragh's lessons in pathophysiology and clinical pearls for treating hypertension. *Am J Hypertens*. 2001;14:491–503.
4. Turnbull F. Blood Pressure Lowering Treatment Trialists' Collaboration. Effects of different blood-pressure-lowering regimens on major cardiovascular events: Results of prospectively-designed overviews of randomized trials. *Lancet*. 2003;362:1527–1535.
5. Wu J, Kraja AT, Oberman A, et al. A summary of the effects of antihypertensive medications on measured blood pressure. *Am J Hypertens*. 2005;18:935–942.
6. Psaty BM, Lumley T, Furberg CD, et al. Health outcomes associated with various antihypertensive therapies used as first-line agents: A network meta-analysis. *JAMA*. 2003;289:2534–2544.
7. ALLHAT Officers and Coordinators for the ALLHAT Collaborative Research Group. Major outcomes in high-risk hypertensive patients randomized to angiotensin-converting enzyme inhibitor or calcium channel blocker vs diuretic: The Antihypertensive and Lipid-Lowering Treatment to Prevent Heart Attack Trial (ALLHAT). *JAMA*. 2002;288:2981–2997.
8. Franse LV, Pahor M, Di Bari M, Somes GW, Cushman WC, Applegate WB. Hypokalemia associated with diuretic use and cardiovascular events in the Systolic Hypertension in the Elderly Program. *Hypertension*. 2000;35:1025–1030.
9. Levine SR, Coull B. Potassium depletion as a risk factor for stroke: Will a banana a day keep your stroke away? *Neurology*. 59;13:302–303.

10. Zimlichman R, Shargorodsky M, Wainstein J. Prolonged treatment of hypertensive patients with low dose HCTZ improves arterial elasticity but not if they have NIDDM or IFG: Treatment with full dose HCTZ (25 mg/d) aggravates metabolic parameters and arterial stiffness. *Am J Hypertens.* 2004;17(suppl 1s):138A.
11. Gress TW, Nieto FJ, Shahar E, Wofford MR, Brancati FL. Hypertension and antihypertensive therapy as risk factors for type 2 diabetes mellitus. *N Engl J Med.* 2000;342:905–912.
12. Kasiske BL, Ma JZ, Kalil RS, Louis TA. Effects of antihypertensive therapy on serum lipids. *Ann Intern Med* 1995;122:133–141.
13. Grimm RH Jr, Grandits GA, Prineas RJ, et al. Long-term effects on sexual function of five antihypertensive drugs and nutritional hygienic treatment in hypertensive men and women: Treatment of Mild Hypertension Study (TOMHS). *Hypertension.* 1997;29:8–14.
14. Choi HK, Atkinson K, Karlson EW, Curhan G. Obesity, weight change, hypertension, diuretic use, and risk of gout in men: The health professionals follow-up study. *Arch Intern Med.* 2005;165:742–748.
15. Sharabi Y, Illan R, Kamari Y, et al. Diuretic induced hyponatremia in elderly hypertensive women. *J Hum Hypertens.* 2002;16:631–635.
16. Dørup I, Skajaa K, Thybo NK. Oral magnesium supplementation restores the concentrations of magnesium, potassium and sodium–potassium pumps in skeletal muscle of patients receiving diuretic treatment. *J Intern Med.* 1993;233:117–123.
17. Psaty BM, Heckbert SR, Koepsell TD, et al. The risk of myocardial infarction associated with antihypertensive drug therapies. *JAMA.* 1995;274:620–625.
18. Furberg CD, Psaty BM, Meyer JV. Nifedipine: Dose-related increase in mortality in patients with coronary heart disease. *Circulation.* 1995;92:1326–1331.
19. Muller JE, Morrison J, Stone PH, et al. Nifedipine therapy for patients with threatened and acute myocardial infarction: A randomized, double-blind, placebo-controlled comparison. *Circulation.* 1984;69:740–747.
20. Nissen SE, Tuzcu EM, Libby P, et al. Effects of antihypertensive agents on cardiovascular events in patients with coronary disease and normal blood pressure: The CAMELOT study: A randomized controlled trial. *JAMA.* 2004;292:2217–2226.
21. Klingbeil AU, Schneider M, Martus P, Messerli FH, Schmieder RE. A meta-analysis of the effects of treatment on left ventricular mass in essential hypertension. *Am J Med.* 2003;115:41–46.
22. Angeli F, Verdecchia P, Reboldi GP, et al. Calcium channel blockade to prevent stroke in hypertension: A meta-analysis of 13 studies with 103,793 subjects. *Am J Hypertens.* 2004;17:817–822.
23. Forette F, Seux ML, Staessen JA, et al. The prevention of dementia with antihypertensive treatment: New evidence from the Systolic Hypertension in Europe (Syst-Eur) Study. *Arch Intern Med.* 2002;162:2046–2052.
24. Van Hamersvelt HW, Kloke HJ, de Jong DJ, Koene RA, Huysmans FT. Oedema formation with the vasodilators nifedipine and diazoxide: Direct local effect or sodium retention? *J Hypertens.* 1996;14:1041–1046.
25. Pahor M, Guralnik JM, Ferrucci L, et al. Calcium-channel blockade and incidence of cancer in aged populations. *Lancet.* 1996;348:493–497.

26. Pahor M, Guralnik JM, Furberg CD, Carbonin P, Havlik R. Risk of gastrointestinal haemorrhage with calcium antagonists in hypertensive persons over 67 years old. *Lancet.* 1996;347:1061–1065.

27. Agodoa LY, Appel L, Bakris GL, et al. Effect of ramipril versus amlodipine on renal outcomes in hypertensive nephrosclerosis: A randomized controlled trial. *JAMA.* 2001;285:2719–2728.

28. Delles C, Klingbeil AU, Schneider MP, Handrock R, Weidinger G, Schmieder RE. Direct comparison of the effects of valsartan and amlodipine on renal hemodynamics in human essential hypertension. *Am J Hypertens.* 2003;16:1030–1035.

29. ALLHAT Collaborative Research Group. Major cardiovascular events in hypertensive patients randomized to doxazosin vs. chlorthalidone: The antihypertensive and lipid-lowering treatment to prevent heart attack trial (ALLHAT). *JAMA.* 2002;288:1967–1975.

30. Stafford RS, Furberg CD, Finkelstein SN, Cockburn IM, Alehegn T, Ma J. Impact of clinical trial results on national trends in α-blocker prescribing, 1996–2002. *JAMA.* 2004;291:54–62.

31. Black HR, Sollins JS, Garofalo JL. The addition of doxazosin to the therapeutic regimen of hypertensive patients inadequately controlled with other antihypertensive medications: A randomized, placebo-controlled study. *Am J Hypertens.* 2000;13:468–474.

32. Kasiske BL, Ma JZ, Kalil RS, Louis TA. Effects of antihypertensive therapy on serum lipids. *Ann Intern Med.* 1995;122:133–141.

33. Lithell HO. Hyperinsulinemia, insulin resistance, and the treatment of hypertension. *Am J Hypertens.* 1996;9:150S–154S.

34. Stokes GS, Graham RM, Gain JM, Davis PR. Influence of dosage and dietary sodium on the first-dose effects of prazosin. *Br Med J.* 1977;1:1507–1508.

35. Marshall HJ, Beevers DG. α-adrenoceptor blocking drugs and female urinary incontinence: Prevalence and reversibility. *Br J Clin Pharmacol.* 1996;42:507–509.

36. Cameron HA, Ramsay LE. The lupus syndrome induced by hydralazine: A common complication with low dose treatment. *Br Med J (Clin Res Ed).* 1984;289:410–412.

37. Nordlander R, Walter M. Once-versus twice-daily administration of controlled-release isosorbide-5-mononitrate 60 mg in treatment of stable angina pectoris: A randomized, double-blind, cross-over study. *Eur Heart J.* 1994;15:108–113.

38. Taylor AL, Ziesches S, Yancy C. Combination of isosorbide dinitrate and hydralazine in blacks with heart failure. *N Engl J Med.* 2004;351:2049–2057.

39. Münzel T, Ziesche S, Yancy C, et al. Hydralazine prevents nitroglycerin tolerance by inhibiting activation of a membrane-bound NADH oxidase: A new action for an old drug. *J Clin Invest.* 1996;98:1465–1470.

40. Sica DA. Minoxidil: An underused vasodilator for resistant or severe hypertension. *J Clin Hypertens.* 2004;6:283–287.

41. Ruggenenti P, Fassi A, Ilieva AP, et al. Preventing microalbuminuria in type 2 diabetes. *N Engl J Med.* 2004;351:1941–1951.

42. Lewis EJ, Hunsicker LG, Bain RP, Rohde RD. The effect of angiotensin-converting-enzyme inhibition on diabetic nephropathy. *N Engl J Med.* 1993;329:1456–1462.

43. The GISEN group (Gruppo Italiano di Studi Epidemioligici in Nefrologia). Randomised placebo-controlled trial of effect of ramipril on decline in glomerular filtration rate and risk of terminal renal failure in proteinuric, nondiabetic nephropathy. *Lancet.* 1997;349:1857–1863.
44. ACE Inhibitor Myocardial Infarction Collaborative Group. Indications for ACE inhibitors in the early treatment of acute myocardial infarction: Systematic overview of individual data from 100,000 patients in randomized trials. *Circulation.* 1998;97:2202–2212.
45. Flather MD, Yusuf S, Køber L, et al. Long-term ACE-inhibitor therapy in patients with heart failure or left-ventricular dysfunction: A systematic overview of data from individual patients. *Lancet.* 2000;355:1575–1581.
46. Croog SH, Levine S, Testa MA, et al. The effects of antihypertensive therapy on the quality of life. *N Engl J Med.* 1986;314:1657–1664.
47. Bakris GL, Weir MR. Angiotensin-converting enzyme inhibitor-associated elevations in serum creatinine: Is this a cause for concern? *Arch Intern Med.* 2000;160:685–693.
48. Johnsen SP, Jacobsen J, Monster TB, Friis S, McLaughlin JK, Sørensen HT. Risk of first-time hospitalization for angioedema among users of ACE inhibitors and angiotensin receptor antagonists. *Am J Med.* 2005;118:1428–1429.
49. Sica DA, Black HR. Current concepts of pharmacotherapy in hypertension: ACE inhibitor-related angioedema: Can angiotensin-receptor blockers be safely used? *J Clin Hypertens.* 2002;4:375–380.
50. Israili ZH, Hall WD. Cough and angioneurotic edema associated with angiotensin-converting enzyme inhibitor therapy: A review of the literature and pathophysiology. *Ann Intern Med.* 1992;117:234–242.
51. Woo KS, Nicholls MG. High prevalence of persistent cough with angiotensin converting enzyme inhibitors in Chinese. *Br J Clin Pharmacol.* 1995;40:141–144.
52. Shotan A, Widerhorn J, Hurst A, Elkayam U. Risks of angiotensin-converting enzyme inhibition during pregnancy: Experimental and clinical evidence, potential mechanisms, and recommendations for use. *Am J Med.* 1994;96:451–456.
53. Fakhouri F, Grünfeld JP, Hermine O, Delarue R. Angiotensin-converting enzyme inhibitors for secondary erythrocytosis. *Ann Int Med.* 2004;140:492–493.
54. Herings RM, de Boer A, Stricker BH, Leufkens HG, Porsius A. Hypoglycaemia associated with use of inhibitors of angiotensin converting enzyme. *Lancet.* 1995;345:1195–1198.
55. Opie LH, Schall R. Old antihypertensives and new diabetes. *J Hypertens.* 2004;22:1453–1458.
56. Conlin PR, Gerth WC, Fox J, Roehm JB, Boccuzzi SJ. Four-year persistence patterns among patients initiating therapy with angiotensin II receptor antagonist losartan versus other antihypertensive drug classes. *Clin Ther.* 2001;23:1999–2010.
57. Lewis EJ, Hunsicker LG, Clarke WR, et al. Renoprotective effect of the angiotensin-receptor antagonist Irbesartan in patients with nephropathy due to type 2 diabetes. *N Engl J Med.* 2001;345:851–860.
58. Devereux RB, Dahlöf B, Kjeldsen SE, et al. Effects of losartan or atenolol in hypertensive patients without clinically evident vascular disease: A substudy of the LIFE randomized trial. *Ann Intern Med.* 2003;139:169–177.

59. Granger CB, McMurray JJ, Yusuf S, et al. Effects of candesartan in patients with chronic heart failure and reduced left-ventricular systolic function intolerant to angiotensin-converting-enzyme inhibitors: The CHARM-Alternative trial. *Lancet*. 2003;362:772–776.

60. Bakris GL, Siomos M, Richardson D, et al. ACE inhibition or angiotensin receptor blockade: Impact on potassium in renal failure. *Kidney Int*. 2000;58:2084–2092.

61. van Rijnsoever EW, Kwee-Zuiderwijk WJ, Feenstra J. Angioneurotic edema attributed to the use of losartan. *Arch Intern Med*. 1998;158:2063–2065.

62. Saji H, Yamanaka M, Hagiwara A, Ijiri R. Losartan and fetal toxic effects. *Lancet*. 2001;357:363.

63. Schupp M, Janke J, Clasen R, Unger T, Kintscher U. Angiotensin type 1 receptor blockers induce peroxisome proliferator-activated receptor-gamma activity. *Circulation*. 2004;109:2054–2057.

64. Oh BH, Mitchell J, Herron JR, Chung J, Khan M, Keefe DL. Aliskirin, an oral renin inhibitor, provides dose-dependant efficacy and sustained 24-hour blood pressure control in patients with hypertension. *J Am Coll Cardiol*. 2007;49:1157–1163.

65. Parving HH, Persson F, Lewis JB, Lewis EJ, Hollenberg NK, AVOID Study Investigators. Aliskiren combined with losaratan in type 2 diabetes and nephropathy. *N Engl J Med*. 2008;358:2433–2446.

66. Solomon SD, Appelbaum E, Manning WJ, et al. Effect of the direct renin inhibitor aliskiren, the angiotensin receptor blocker losartan, or both on left ventricular mass in patients with left ventricular hypertrophy. *Circulation*. 2009;119:530–537.

67. Gradman AH, Schmieder RE, Lins RL, Nussberger J, Chiang Y, Bedigian MP. Aliskiren, a novel orally effective inhibitor, provides dose-dependent anti-hypertensive efficacy and placebo-like tolerability in hypertensive patients. *Circulation*. 2005;111:1012–1018.

68. Messerli FH, Beevers DG, Franklin SS, Pickering TG. Beta-blockers in hypertension—The emperor has no clothes: An open letter to present and prospective drafters of new guidelines for the treatment of hypertension. *Am J Hypertens*. 2003;16:870–873.

69. Carlberg B, Samuelsson O, Lindholm LH. Atenolol in hypertension: Is it a wise choice? *Lancet*. 2004;364:1684–1689.

70. The Norwegian Multicenter Study Group. Timolol-induced reduction in mortality and reinfarction in patients surviving acute myocardial infarction. *N Engl J Med*. 1981;304:801–807.

71. The Cardiac Insufficiency Bisoprolol Study II (CIBIS-II): A randomized trial. *Lancet*. 1999;353:9–13.

72. Lindenauer PK, Fitzgerald J, Hoople N, Benjamin EM. The potential preventability of postoperative myocardial infarction. Underuse of perioperative beta-adrenergic blockade. *Arch Intern Med*. 2004;164:762–766.

73. Psaty BM, Koepsell TD, Wagner EH, LoGerfo JP, Inui TS. The relative risk of incident coronary heart disease associated with recently stopping the use of beta-blockers. *JAMA*. 1990;263:1653–1657.

74. Salpeter SR, Ormiston TM, Salpeter EE. Cardioselective beta-blockers in patients with reactive airway disease: A meta-analysis. *Ann Intern Med*. 2002;137:715–725.

75. Gress TW, Nieto FJ, Shahar E, Wofford MR, Brancati FL. Hypertension and antihypertensive therapy as risk factors for type 2 diabetes mellitus. *N Engl J Med*. 2000;342:905–912.

76. Kasiske BL, Ma JZ, Kalil RS, Louis TA. Effects of antihypertensive therapy on serum lipids. *Ann Intern Med*. 1995;122:133–141.

77. Vanhees L, Defoor JG, Schepers D, et al. Effect of bisoprolol and atenolol on endurance exercise capacity in healthy men. *J Hypertens*. 2000;18:35–43.

78. Byrd BF 3rd, Collins HW, Primm RK. Risk factors for severe bradycardia during oral clonidine therapy for hypertension. *Arch Intern Med*. 1988;148:729–733.

79. Rodman JS, Deutsch DJ, Gutman SI. Methyldopa hepatitis: A report of six cases and review of the literature. *Am J Med*. 1976;60:941–948.

80. Neusy AJ, Lowenstein J. Blood pressure and blood pressure variability following withdrawal of propanolol and clonidine. *J Clin Pharmacol*. 1989;29:18–24.

81. Houston MC. Treatment of hypertensive emergencies and urgencies with oral clonidine loading and titration: A review. *Arch Intern Med*. 1986;146:586–589.

82. Bond WS. Psychiatric indications for clonidine: The neuropharmacologic and clinical basis. *J Clin Psychopharmacol*. 1986;6:81–87.

83. Pandya KJ, Raubertas RF, Flynn PJ, et al. Oral clonidine in postmenopausal patients with breast cancer experiencing tamoxifen-induced hot flashes: A University of Rochester Cancer Center Community Clinical Oncology Program study. *Ann Intern Med*. 2000;132:788–793.

84. Cohn JN, Pfeffer MA, Rouleau J, et al. Adverse mortality effect of central sympathetic inhibition with sustained-release moxonidine in patients with heart failure (MOXCON). *Eur J Heart Fail*. 2003;5:659–667.

chapter five

Nutrition

Lifestyle modification is an important part of hypertension management and of overall health. There are several well-accepted comprehensive guidelines that meticulously describe the measures of a healthy lifestyle. They include direction in eating a healthy and balanced diet, maintaining a normal body weight, engaging in adequate physical activity, and minimizing harmful habits and addictions. Two examples of these are the Dietary Guidelines for Americans[1] from the U.S. Department of Agriculture and U.S. Department of Health and Human Services, and the National Cholesterol Education Program (NCEP)[2] from the National Heart, Lung, and Blood Institute of the National Institutes of Health. These guidelines promote the acquisition of adequate dietary nutrients with preference to consumption of unprocessed foods such as fruits, vegetables, and whole grains, a diet similar to that of prehistoric man. The recommendations rely on advice from the Institute of Medicine, which is a nonprofit and nongovernmental American organization, as well as current research and clinical studies. Nutrients can be divided into micronutrients (such as vitamins and minerals) and macronutrients (the calorie-based food groups such as fats, carbohydrates, proteins, and fiber). The Institute of Medicine provides Dietary Reference Intakes (DRIs) for most nutrients, comprised of a set of values defining the recommended daily amounts as well as the safe ranges.[3] This chapter will focus on several nutrients that affect blood pressure without prejudice to others essential to overall health.

The DRIs guide health care governing bodies, nutritionists, and health care providers in advising on adequate nutritional intake. The Recommended Dietary Allowance (RDA), the Adequate Intake (AI), and the Tolerable Upper Intake Level (UL) together help define the amounts of each essential nutrient needed to sustain health. For example, they may suggest the appropriate daily intake of vitamin D, folic acid, protein, and so on. They apply only to healthy people and should not be used in individuals with acute or chronic illness or with nutritional deficiencies. It is an impressive work that combines scientific research and statistical analysis to best estimate these needs. The DRIs are separated into various groups classified according to age, gender, and physiologic state—such as pregnant women, male or female children ages 1 to 3 years, male or female middle-aged people—which all have different needs. The suggested intake levels are applicable to practically all those within each group and each has a reference height and weight, representing the median (or typical) individual. For example, the reference height for adult males is 178 cm (70 inches) and the reference weight is 70 kg (154 pounds), whereas the corresponding values in adult females are 163 cm (64 inches) and 57 kg (126 pounds). Despite a centering of values around reference sizes, which clearly vary within a population, the suggested intakes still pertain to most people within a group. Of course, some discretion must be used for extreme outliers, such as the 2.1 m (7 foot) tall basketball player or the 1.2 m (4 foot) tall gymnast. The RDA represents the average daily nutrient intake level sufficient to meet the nutritional requirements of nearly all (97%–98%) healthy individuals in a particular life stage and gender group.[3] The AI is the recommended average daily intake level assumed to be adequate, based on observed or experimentally determined estimates of nutrient intake by apparently healthy people.[3] These estimates are used because, unlike the RDA, there is limited available scientific evidence to support the AI values. The UL is the highest average daily nutrient intake level that is unlikely to pose risk of adverse health effects.[3] The DRIs, therefore, provide the adequate intake levels of essential nutrients and their upper limits of safety.

The last important term is the Acceptable Macronutrient Distribution Range (AMDR), which is used for calorie- (or energy-) based nutrients: carbohydrates, fats, and proteins. The AMDR is the range of intakes of an energy source associated with a reduced risk of chronic disease that can provide adequate amounts of essential nutrients.[3] For example, the AMDR of carbohydrates for adults and children of both genders is 45%–65% of the total calorie intake. The Dietary Guidelines for Americans formulates its dietary recommendations largely on the DRIs provided by the Institute of Medicine. Although these guidelines are quite comprehensive, their purpose is not to create specific diet plans but rather to present the framework of a healthy lifestyle by incorporating wholesome and healthy foods. However, they do endorse several popular eating plans such as the Dietary Approaches to Stop Hypertension (DASH) eating plan and the USDA Food Patterns. These are simple enough to allow an individual to design an appropriate meal plan, although assistance from a nutritionist is helpful. Although there are more aggressive dietary and lifestyle modification plans available that claim and often do provide quicker results in achieving target weight loss and lower cholesterol levels, the slower and more balanced approach seems safer.

Micronutrients

Sodium (salt) reduction

The influence of dietary sodium (salt) on blood pressure is well regarded and time honored. This relationship was recognized as far back as the era of Emperor Haung Ti, over 4000 years ago. Prehistoric man existed on a diet mostly composed of fruits, nuts, legumes, and some animal products—the so called hunter-gatherer diet—which had a modest sodium intake of about 770 mg (33 mEq) a day.[4] This is substantially less than the typical Western diet, which contains over 3000 mg (130 mEq) of sodium a day[5] with more than 75% coming from nondiscretionary sources such as added preservatives and flavor enhancers. Observational studies of "low-salt" societies show practically no hypertension, compared with a rate of about 30% in Western societies. One such example is in the Yanomamo Indians of the Amazon rain forest basin, who consume about 25 mg (1 mEq) of sodium each day, and hypertension is nonexistent among the more than 500 tribe members.[6] Another interesting study notes that Kenyan Luo tribe members who migrated to the Kenyan capital of Nairobi showed a significant rise in blood pressure compared with tribe members who remained in their ancestral rural setting.[7] A change from a low- to high-sodium diet was thought to be a prime contributor to this effect, although other factors such as the stresses of city life also must be considered. There appears to be a set point between 1150 and 2300 mg (50 to 100 mEq) of daily sodium intake in which salt-mediated hypertension manifests.[8] Ironically, the Dietary Reference Tolerable Upper Intake Level (DRI/UL) is 2300 mg (100 mEq or 1 teaspoon of salt),[3] but this rather high value is likely due to the unfortunate reality of the pervasiveness of sodium in the Western diet. The Dietary Reference Adequate Intake (DRI/AI) level of 1500 mg for adults up to 50 years, 1300 mg for those 51 to 70 years, and 1200 mg for those over 70 years is likely more appropriate, especially for people with hypertension. In most individuals, lowering sodium intake to 2300 mg (100 mEq) per day would result in only a modest decrease in blood pressure, whereas further reduction to about 1150 mg (50 mEq) would more significantly lower blood pressure. There is even evidence that excess sodium imparts a lasting effect on blood pressure that may start very early in life, and this effect may not be entirely reversible with subsequent intake reduction. A study of newborn Dutch infants compared a low-sodium to a normal-sodium diet for the first 6 months of life and showed a systolic blood pressure lower by 2.1 mm Hg in the former group.[9] When these children were examined 15 years later, their systolic blood pressure was still lower by 3.6 mm Hg, despite consuming equivalent diets.[10] The well-publicized Intersalt study compared different societies worldwide and found more elevated blood pressure in people who chronically consume higher levels of sodium.[11] It also suggests an irreversible component despite reducing sodium intake later in life.

Although the effect of excess sodium ingestion is clearly important in the development of hypertension, the corollary effect of a low-sodium diet on lowering blood pressure is not quite as expected. Many large studies show only a modest decrease of systolic/diastolic blood pressure of 4–6/1–3 mm Hg in people with hypertension and 1–2/0–1 mm

Hg in people without hypertension for every 2300 mg (100 mEq) daily reduction.[12-14] However, these studies represent the entire population and when focus is shifted to the elderly subgroup, who more commonly have hypertension, the effect appears to be greater. In this group, there may be a decrease in systolic/diastolic blood pressure of 10/5 mm Hg for every 2300 mg (100 mEq) daily reduction in sodium.[15] This is probably due to an increase in salt sensitivity with age. A low-salt diet is a V (volume)-type method of lowering blood pressure.

Despite the clear cause-and-effect relationship between excess sodium and elevated blood pressure, there is debate, often raucous, about the overall harmful effects of a high-sodium diet. Despite considerable evidence that such a diet is associated with pathology such as ventricular hypertrophy, kidney disease, stroke,[16] and kidney stones,[17] there is seemingly contradictory evidence suggesting that people with hypertension who consume less sodium are more prone to heart attacks.[18] In contrast, people across the entire population who consume less salt have higher mortality rates, particularly from cardiovascular disease.[19] Furthermore, low-salt societies, such as the Yanomamo Indians, appear to have rather short lifespans, with only 5% of the tribe members living beyond 50 years, in clear contrast to the longevity of Western society. It may be relevant that their plasma renin levels also are elevated, as typically seen in reduced-salt diets,[20] because elevated renin and angiotensin II levels are associated with atherosclerosis, heart disease, and stroke.[21] A possible explanation for these seemingly contradictory effects of a reduced-sodium diet (i.e., reducing blood pressure yet increasing mortality rates) may be related to the initial blood pressure of the study populations. Clearly, both elevated blood pressure and higher renin and angiotensin II levels are mediators of cardiovascular disease and stroke. Many of the studies that suggest a poor health outcome of a low-sodium diet compare people who either do not have hypertension or who have treated and controlled hypertension. Because the blood pressure in these groups is probably not significantly affected by the amount of sodium in the diet, it is logical to expect that those with higher renin and angiotensin II levels will be less healthy. Given all of this seemingly contradictory outcomes data, a modest reduction of sodium intake to less than 2300 mg (100 mEq) per day makes sense in the general population, as suggested in the Dietary Guidelines for Americans. However, intake of 1500 mg (65 mEq) or less should be considered in people with hypertension or in those predisposed to hypertension such as black people, middle-aged and older people, and people with diabetes or kidney disease.

Potassium

Although sodium intake is often considered the primary dietary factor in the genesis of hypertension, many believe that potassium intake is equally or perhaps even more important. As with sodium, there is a considerable difference in potassium intake in the typical Western diet compared with that of prehistoric man. However, unlike the increased patterns of sodium intake in the former, potassium intake is far lower than that of prehistoric man or of present day uncultured hunter-gatherer societies. It is estimated that the late Paleolithic diet contained about 10,500 mg (270 mEq) of potassium a day[4] compared with about 2700 mg (69 mEq) in Western society.[22] Epidemiologic studies, such as the National Health and Nutritional Examination Survey III (NHANES III), which follows health-related trends in the United States, suggest an association of high-potassium diets with lower blood pressure.[22] An interesting study in the 1950s in the Akita prefecture of northern Japan compared the diets of two sociologically similar villages having different average blood pressures. Investigators found that villagers in both venues consumed a similar traditional high-salt Japanese diet, but the village with the higher blood pressure consumed less potassium. To test the hypothesis that potassium intake is associated with blood pressure, villagers from the low-potassium community increased their potassium intake by adding 8 to 10 apples a day, with resultant lowering of their blood pressure.[23] Although this study has many uncontrolled variables to explain this effect—for example, the total sodium content of their diet might have decreased due to substituting typical foods with apples—the study focused attention on the contribution of potassium to blood pressure, resulting in numerous other controlled studies. Many attribute the higher incidence of hypertension among black communities in the United States to a low-potassium diet.[24] A more recent study of Japanese people with hypertension showed a modest reduction in blood pressure with daily supplementation with 2500 mg (64 mEq) of slow-release potassium.[25] A typical response to a 2340 mg (60 mEq) potassium supplement in people with hypertension is a reduction in systolic/diastolic blood pressure of 3–7/1–4 mm Hg.[26,27]

Surprisingly, there are few studies of potassium intake and its effect on cardiovascular disease. Observational studies, such as those involving the Yanomamo Indians, suggest a protective effect of a high-potassium diet, as there is no significant cardiovascular disease in such societies compared with Western society.[6] Other studies suggest a high-potassium diet is preventative of stroke,[28,29] and animal studies show protection from hypertensive kidney disease.[30] This effect for both stroke and renal disease may be related to less atherosclerosis and improved endothelial function. The mechanisms by which potassium intake lowers blood pressure is largely due to a diuretic effect and a direct inhibition of renin production by the kidneys.[31,32] The diuretic effect may be so large as to cause a compensatory stimulation of renin production, resulting in increased overall renin levels in some people. As such, a high potassium intake is a mixed R (renin)- and V-type method of lowering blood pressure.

The DRI/AI of potassium is 4700 mg (121 mEq) per day,[3] and ingestion of this amount would probably help lower blood pressure. Dietary means to achieve this level are preferable, although potassium supplements can be considered. However, caution should be heeded, especially in those with kidney disease, as they have limited ability to regulate potassium balance and may become potassium toxic. Slow-release potassium tablets are commercially available, although there are many preferable dietary sources rich in potassium. Table 5.1 lists several potassium-rich foods and their potassium content.

Table 5.1 Common Potassium-Rich Foods

Food item	Potassium content	Serving size
Tuna	484 mg, 12 mEq	3 ounces, 85 grams
Dried apricots	407 mg, 10 mEq	10 pieces, 35 grams
Avocado	144 mg, 4 mEq	1 ounce, 28 grams
Banana	422 mg, 11 mEq	1 medium, 118 grams
Dates	542 mg, 14 mEq	5 pieces, 42 grams
Cantaloupe	272 mg, 7 mEq	1 cup, 160 grams
Orange	161 mg, 4 mEq	1 medium, 110 grams
Raisins	1086 mg, 27 mEq	1 cup, 145 grams
Carrot juice	689 mg, 18 mEq	1 cup, 236 grams
Orange juice	496 mg, 13 mEq	1 cup, 248 grams
Prune juice	707 mg, 18 mEq	1 cup, 256 grams
Tomato juice	556 mg, 14 mEq	1 cup, 243 grams
Low-fat yogurt	531 mg, 14 mEq	8 ounces, 227 grams
Almonds	200 mg, 5 mEq	1 ounce, 28 grams
Baked beans	569 mg, 14 mEq	1 cup, 254 grams
Kidney beans (cooked)	713 mg, 18 mEq	1 cup, 177 grams
Pinto beans (cooked)	746 mg, 19 mEq	1 cup, 171 grams
White beans	1189 mg, 30 mEq	1 cup, 262 grams
Broccoli (cooked)	457 mg, 12 mEq	1 cup, 156 grams
Brussels sprouts (cooked)	495 mg, 12 mEq	1 cup, 156 grams
Chick peas (cooked)	477 mg, 12 mEq	1 cup, 164 grams
Lentils (cooked)	731 mg, 18 mEq	1 cup, 198 grams
Soybeans (cooked)	886 mg, 23 mEq	1 cup, 172 grams
Spinach (cooked)	839 mg, 22 mEq	1 cup, 180 grams
Winter squash (cooked)	494 mg, 12 mEq	1 cup, 205 grams
Sweet potato (baked/skin)	694 mg, 17 mEq	1 cup, 146 grams
Potato (baked with skin)	1081 mg, 28 mEq	1 potato, 202 grams
Raw tomato	427 mg, 11 mEq	1 cup, 180 grams

Calcium

Calcium intake in a modern Western diet differs from the hunter-gatherer diet of prehistoric times; today's typical diet contains about 760 mg (19 mmol) of calcium each day[22] compared with 2000 mg (50 mmol) in prehistoric times.[4] Only 25% to 50% of ingested calcium is absorbed in the gastrointestinal tract, with the remainder excreted in stool. Body calcium levels are tightly controlled by vitamin D and parathyroid hormone; vitamin D primarily regulates intestinal absorption, whereas parathyroid hormone helps maintain steady blood levels. Daily calcium supplementation of 1200 mg (30 mmol), which is above typical dietary intake, is associated with a small reduction in systolic/diastolic blood pressure of 1–2/0–1 mm Hg.[33,34] This effect may be slightly higher in people with hypertension. There also is an association between body weight and calcium intake. Studies suggest body weight is reduced by as much as 8 kg (17 pounds) for each 1000 mg per day increase in daily calcium consumption.[35] A lower body weight also may contribute to a lower blood pressure. The mechanism whereby a low-calcium diet causes blood pressure elevation and weight gain may be associated with alterations in parathyroid hormone and vitamin D levels, as the body increases production of both in response to calcium deficiency. Parathyroid hormone is associated with increased blood pressure,[36] an effect partially mediated by increased renin secretion and subsequent activation of the renin–angiotensin system (RAS).[37] Parathyroid hormone also may slow the basal metabolic rate, which could explain the higher weights of people on lower-calcium diets.[35] This effect may have been protective in prior times when famine was common, causing deficiency of all nutrients, including calcium. Subsequent elevated parathyroid hormone levels and consequent lower metabolic rates may have preserved body fat and muscle mass. Overall, calcium intake has only a modest effect on lowering blood pressure, although dietary intake of low-fat dairy products (commonly associated with calcium intake) seems to have a more prominent effect as shown in the DASH diet.[38] However, dairy products are a mix of substances, including vitamin D and various proteins, which may also affect the blood pressure. Because calcium inhibits renin production,[39,40] its supplementation is an R-type method of lowering blood pressure.

The DRI/RDA for calcium is 1000 mg per day for adult women ≤50 years old, 1200 mg for women >50 years old, 1000 mg for adult men ≤70 years old, and 1200 mg for men >70 years old.[3] The National Osteoporosis Foundation adopts these recommendations and the DASH diet provides for similar amounts. Table 5.2 lists several calcium-rich foods and their respective calcium content.

Table 5.2 Common Calcium-Rich Foods

Food item	Calcium content	Serving size
Sardines	325 mg, 8 mmol	3 ounces, 85 grams
Rhubarb (cooked)	348 mg, 9 mmol	1 cup, 240 grams
Collards (cooked)	266 mg, 7 mmol	1 cup, 190 grams
Soybeans (cooked)	261 mg, 7 mmol	1 cup, 180 grams
Spinach (cooked)	245 mg, 6 mmol	1 cup, 180 grams
Ricotta cheese	669 mg, 17 mmol	1 cup, 246 grams
Yogurt (low fat)	415 mg, 10 mmol	8 ounces, 227 grams
Milk (low fat)	290 mg, 7 mmol	1 cup, 244 grams
Swiss cheese	224 mg, 6 mmol	1 ounce, 28 grams
Mozzarella (cheese)	207 mg, 5 mmol	1 ounce, 28 grams
Muenster (cheese)	203 mg, 5 mmol	1 ounce, 28 grams
Tofu	133 mg, 4 mmol	1 piece, 120 grams

Magnesium

Magnesium is an important nutrient with diverse effects. It is found in bone, helps regulate muscle and nerve activity, and is involved in many chemical reactions in the body. As with the aforementioned minerals, magnesium intake in the modern Western diet also significantly differs from that of the hunter-gatherer diet of prehistoric times. A typical Western diet contains about 280 mg (12 mmol) of magnesium per day[22] compared with 800 mg (33 mmol) in a natural diet similar to that of prehistoric times.[41] Only 40% to 50% of ingested magnesium is absorbed in the gastrointestinal tract. To maintain homeostasis, most absorbed magnesium is excreted in the urine with some also excreted in stool and sweat. Although vitamin D has a small role in regulating absorption rates, it is mostly independent of regulating hormones. Observational studies suggest an association between a low-magnesium diet and hypertension,[42] although the corollary effect of dietary magnesium supplementation in lowering blood pressure is controversial. A meta-analysis of 20 independent studies suggests a modest decrease in systolic/diastolic blood pressure of 1/1 mm Hg with magnesium supplementation.[43] However, many of the studies included in this analysis had large changes in blood pressure in both a positive and negative direction. A more pronounced effect occurs in people with hypertension[44] and in those with deficient stores of magnesium,[45] which is common with diuretic use. The effect is greater with high doses of supplements, typically 480 to 960 mg (20–40 mmol) per day. The mechanism by which magnesium lowers blood pressure involves a blockade of the calcium channels of the arteriolar smooth muscle cells.[46] As described in Chapter 4, calcium influx into these cells causes vasoconstriction and subsequent blood pressure elevation. Magnesium blocks these channels and prevents this process, effectively acting as a calcium channel blocker. A secondary effect occurs by blocking the calcium channels in nerve endings, which inhibits the release of norepinephrine[47] and subsequently limits constriction of the blood vessels. Magnesium supplementation is therefore a V-type method of lowering blood pressure. Magnesium also affects renal potassium regulation by an uncertain mechanism, and magnesium deficiency is associated with urinary wasting of potassium. It is difficult to correct blood potassium deficits without first correcting the magnesium deficit, so both elements are often given together.[48] Perhaps potassium deficiency also contributes to higher blood pressure in people with magnesium deficiency.

Despite the suggested Dietary Reference Intake/Recommended Dietary Allowance (DRI/RDA) of 420 mg (18 mmol) of magnesium per day for men over 30 years old and 320 (13 mmol) mg for women over 30 years old,[3] higher levels seem reasonable in treating hypertension. However, caution must be exercised, especially in those with kidney disease, as these individuals have limited ability to regulate magnesium homeostasis and excretion. Dietary sources of magnesium are preferable but commercially available slow-release magnesium tablets can be considered too. Table 5.3 lists several magnesium-rich foods and their magnesium content.

Vitamin D and parathyroid hormone

Although vitamin D and parathyroid hormone were once thought to only regulate calcium and phosphorus homeostasis, broader effects are now appreciated. Vitamin D and parathyroid hormone are intricately connected, as they carefully regulate each other's level and effect. Because their function is complicated, it is best described with the aid of a diagram (Figure 5.1). In humans, total vitamin D levels are comprised of two active forms—vitamin D3 (cholecalciferol) and vitamin D2 (ergocalciferol)—and typical laboratory testing includes a breakdown into these components. Vitamin D3 is mostly produced in animals, whereas vitamin D2 comes from plants and fungi. In humans, vitamin D3 is primarily synthesized in the skin from its precursor compound, provitamin D, although some is obtained from the diet and through supplements. In contrast, vitamin D2 is obtained from the diet and supplements only. Natural foods are somewhat limited in vitamin D content, so most dietary intake comes in either pill/liquid form or from fortified foods. Fatty fish, eggs, liver, and some mushrooms are examples of natural sources, and milk, breads, and cereals are common fortified sources. Studies from the 1930s suggested equivalent health benefits from both forms of vitamin D, although this finding has been challenged more recently with a belief that vitamin D3 is superior. For historical reasons, only vitamin D2 has pharmacologic status in the United States and is the form commonly prescribed by physicians,

Table 5.3 Common Magnesium-Rich Foods

Food item	Magnesium content	Serving size
Halibut	91 mg, 3.8 mmol	3 ounces, 85 grams
Tuna	54 mg, 2.25 mmol	3 ounces, 85 grams
Artichokes	50 mg, 2.1 mmol	1 medium, 120 grams
Banana	32 mg, 1.3 mmol	1 medium, 118 grams
Dried figs	26 mg, 1.1 mmol	2 pieces, 38 grams
Prune juice	36 mg, 1.5 mmol	1 cup, 256 grams
Whole milk	24 mg, 1.0 mmol	1 cup, 244 grams
Low-fat yogurt	39 mg, 1.6 mmol	8 ounces, 227 grams
Almonds	76 mg, 3.2 mmol	1 ounce, 28 grams
Cashews	74 mg, 3.1 mmol	1 ounce, 28 grams
Pine nuts	71 mg, 3.0 mmol	1 ounce, 28 grams
Brazil nuts	107 mg, 4.5 mmol	1 ounce, 28 grams
Baked beans	69 mg, 2.9 mmol	1 cup, 254 grams
White beans	134 mg, 5.6 mmol	1 cup, 262 grams
Black beans (cooked)	120 mg, 5.0 mmol	1 cup, 172 grams
Navy beans (cooked)	96 mg, 4.0 mmol	1 cup, 182 grams
Broccoli (cooked)	33 mg, 1.4 mmol	1 cup, 156 grams
Spinach (cooked)	157 mg, 6.5 mmol	1 cup, 180 grams
Soybeans (cooked)	148 mg, 6.2 mmol	1 cup, 172 grams
Chickpeas (cooked)	79 mg, 3.3 mmol	1 cup, 164 grams
Pumpkin seeds	156 mg, 6.5 mmol	1 ounce, 28 grams
Okra (cooked)	94 mg, 3.9 mmol	1 cup, 184 grams
Lentils (cooked)	71 mg, 3.0 mmol	1 cup, 198 grams
Tomato paste	134 mg, 5.6 mmol	1 cup, 262 grams
Potatoes (with skin)	57 mg, 2.4 mmol	1 potato, 202 grams
Barley	158 mg, 6.6 mmol	1 cup, 200 grams
Buckwheat flour	301 mg, 12.5 mmol	1 cup, 120 grams
Oat bran	221 mg, 9.2 mmol	1 cup, 94 grams
Wheat flour	166 mg, 6.9 mmol	1 cup, 120 grams
Cornmeal	155 mg, 6.6 mmol	1 cup, 138 grams

although vitamin D3 is available as an over-the-counter product. One important difference is that the megadose form of 1250 µg (50,000 IU), which can be conveniently taken weekly or monthly instead of smaller daily doses, is mostly available in the vitamin D2 form, although higher doses of vitamin D3 are now offered on the Internet and in some pharmacies, too. Vitamin D itself is a relatively inactive compound but is converted to the active form, 1,25-dihydroxyvitamin D (calcitriol) by sequential hydroxylation in the liver and kidneys (Figure 5.1). This compound

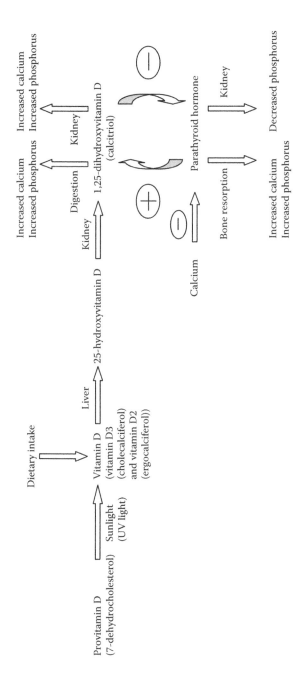

Figure 5.1 Schematic of vitamin D and parathyroid hormone metabolism.

increases calcium and phosphorus levels by promoting absorption in the digestive tract and by minimizing kidney excretion in urine.

Parathyroid hormone is produced primarily by the parathyroid gland and promotes bone resorption, causing release of bone calcium and phosphorus into the blood. It also inhibits urinary calcium excretion while enhancing urinary phosphorus excretion (Figure 5.1). This hormone raises blood levels of calcium but lowers phosphorus levels as the urinary phosphorus excretion component outweighs bone resorption. The two hormones are tightly regulated by a feedback mechanism, whereby parathyroid hormone promotes 1,25-dihydroxyvitamin D production but 1,25-dihydroxyvitamin D feeds back to diminish parathyroid hormone production (Figure 5.1). Calcium also inhibits parathyroid hormone production (Figure 5.1). Calcium and to some degree phosphorus blood levels are very tightly regulated by this system.

It is difficult to discuss the role of vitamin D in health independently of parathyroid hormone. Cross-sectional and prospective studies show an association of vitamin D deficiency with cardiovascular disease,[49–51] stroke,[52] and all-cause mortality.[53] Blood glucose regulation is also affected, as insulin resistance, metabolic syndrome,[54] and diabetes[55] positively correlate with vitamin D deficiency. Similar findings occur with elevated parathyroid hormone levels, which also positively correlate with cardiovascular disease,[56,57] insulin resistance,[58] and metabolic syndrome.[59] Vitamin D deficiency also is associated with elevated blood pressure.[60,61] Studies with black people suggest that their prevalence of hypertension may be due in part to low levels of vitamin D.[62] Disproportionately higher rates of hypertension during winter months compared with summer months and in populations farther from the equator also may be due to varying levels of vitamin D as a function of sunshine and ultraviolet light exposure.[63] Vitamin D deficiency is also predictive of future development of hypertension.[64] Higher parathyroid hormone levels are similarly associated with elevated blood pressure[65,66] and with future development of hypertension.[67]

Despite a strong relationship between low vitamin D levels and elevated blood pressure, the corollary expectation that vitamin D intake, through either natural dietary means or supplements, can lower blood pressure has not been clearly established. Although some studies suggest a blood-pressure-lowering effect with increased vitamin D intake,[68,69] others do not.[70] Of interest, low-fat dairy products, which are high in vitamin D, are associated with lower blood pressure, although these foods contain other active substances such as calcium and various proteins that may contribute to the effect.[71] No cardiovascular disease benefit is clearly evident with vitamin D supplementation.[72] A deeper explanation of the function of vitamin D and parathyroid hormone may help explain these seemingly contradictory effects (Figure 5.2). There is a direct relationship between these hormones and the RAS, as vitamin D suppresses and

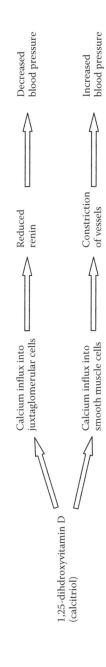

Figure 5.2 Effect of 1,25-dihydroxyvitamin D on blood pressure.

parathyroid hormone enhances renin production in the kidneys.[73] This occurs as vitamin D influences intracellular calcium levels of the juxta-glomerular cells of the kidneys by regulating the calcium channels of the cell walls. Calcitriol opens these channels, allowing calcium influx and subsequent suppression of renin gene expression.[74,75] As such, vita-min D supplementation should be more useful in treating people with renin-mediated hypertension. However, other cell types, such as the vas-cular smooth muscle cells, are similarly affected, and influx of calcium into these cells would cause constriction of the vessels and blood pressure elevation.[76] These opposing effects of lowering renin levels and increasing vascular resistance may explain some of the discrepancy observed in the literature. Calcitriol also is produced by white blood cell macrophages, which, unlike production in the kidneys, occurs in an unregulated man-ner. Macrophages are part of atherosclerotic plaque, so high levels of cal-citriol can be produced locally in blood vessels, especially in individuals with vascular disease. Aside from raising blood pressure, high levels have the potential to promote unregulated inflammation, endothelial dysfunc-tion, and further propagation of atherosclerosis.[77,78]

There appears to be a bimodal effect whereby both low and high lev-els of vitamin D have adverse health effects. A study comparing all-cause mortality rates and vitamin D levels shows an optimal blood level range of 25-hydroxyvitamin D between 30 and 49 ng/mL.[53] Mortality rates are increased in people with both lower and higher levels, possibly due to higher renin levels in those with lower levels and increased inflamma-tion and endothelial dysfunction in those with higher levels. There is no absolute consensus as to normal blood levels of 25-hydroxyvitamin D, but most authorities consider a level of 30 ng/mL or above to be adequate.[79] Vitamin D insufficiency is usually defined at a level between 20 and 29 ng/mL and deficiency at levels <20 ng/mL. Based on these definitions, there is some concern that 30% to 50% of the general population may have low vitamin D stores.[80]

In 2011, the Institute of Medicine revised its recommendations for vitamin D intake at the request of the United States and Canadian govern-ments, as a swell of new data and public sentiment favored higher levels. The DRI/RDA of vitamin D is 15 µg (600 IU) per day in adult men and women between ages 18 and 70 years, and 20 µg (800 IU) in those over 70 years.[81] The DRI/UL for all adults is 100 µg (4000 IU) per day. These modest doses should maintain blood levels of 25-hydroxyvitamin D of at least 20 ng/dL, which is considered sufficient by the Institute of Medicine. Many feel these levels are still too low and higher levels have been sug-gested. Daily megadoses have been advocated, although caution must be used as such levels may cause harmful effects such as systemic inflam-mation, endothelial dysfunction, and potentially elevated blood pressure. A reasonable approach is to target the 25-hydroxyvitamin D blood level

Table 5.4 Common Vitamin-D-Rich Foods

Food item	Vitamin D content	Serving size
Salmon, sockeye	19.8 µg, 792 IU	3 ounces, 85 grams
Milk, whole (with added vitamin D)	3.2 µg, 128 IU	1 cup
Milk, 1% (with added vitamin D)	2.9 µg, 116 IU	1 cup
Cheese, ricotta	0.5 µg, 20 IU	1 medium, 118 grams
Egg, whole	0.7 µg, 28 IU	1 extra large
Mushrooms, shiitake	1.2 µg, 48 IU	1 cup

to 30 to 49 ng/mL. In people with vitamin D deficiency, weekly doses of 1250 µg (50,000 IU) of vitamin D for 6 to 8 weeks and then daily doses of 20 to 25 µg (800–1000 IU) are suggested. In those with vitamin D insufficiency, daily intake of 20 to 25 µg (800–1000 IU) is suggested. After 3 months, the 25-hydroxyvitamin D level should be rechecked and adjusted accordingly. The 25-hydroxyvitamin D blood level should be checked in all people with hypertension. No supplementation may be needed in individuals with adequate levels as they may be receiving sufficient amounts through their diet and through sun/ultraviolet exposure. If levels are low, it is reasonable to aggressively replete the stores to adequate levels. However, given the complexity of this topic as well as the potential for harmful side effects with elevated levels, it is difficult to suggest levels higher than standard doses. As vitamin D supplementation reduces renin production, it is considered an R-type method of lowering blood pressure. Table 5.4 lists several foods with high vitamin D content.

Vitamin C (ascorbic acid)

Vitamin C is an important nutrient involved in the growth and repair of body tissue. It regulates the synthesis of collagen, the main protein of connective tissue. Vitamin C deficiency causes scurvy, which is still present in some industrialized countries. Adequate intake is probably protective against cardiovascular disease and cancer[82] and may prevent eye diseases such as cataracts and macular degeneration.[83] There is speculation about its ability to boost the immune system and some think it can even prevent the common cold.[84] It may improve diabetes as well.[85] Linus Pauling, the famous scientist and statesman, was a strong advocate of high doses of vitamin C. Toward the end of his life, he reportedly took up to 18 g a day. (I had the opportunity to hear him speak when he was 92 years old and he was still witty and lucid. Who can argue with a two-time Nobel Prize laureate?) Typical daily intake of vitamin C in a modern Western diet is about 80 to 110 mg compared with about 600 mg in the prehistoric hunter-gatherer diet.[4] Observational studies confirm an association between higher vitamin C dietary intake and lower blood pressure.[86] Several relatively small studies have analyzed the effects of vitamin C supplementation on blood pressure and most have shown reduction. Unfortunately, there is no large and conclusive study, but an average response in people with hypertension is a decrease in systolic/diastolic blood pressure of 4/2 mm Hg.[87] Larger reductions are expected in people with endothelial dysfunction such as diabetes.[88] Vitamin C acts by improving endothelial dysfunction primarily through its antioxidant effects. It scavenges for harmful free radicals, minimizing their effects on promoting atherosclerosis, arterial stiffness, and consequent hypertension.[89–91] A secondary mechanism involves stabilization of the nutrient tetrahydrobiopterin (THB), which is a cofactor for the enzyme that produces nitric oxide. Increased levels of THB directly increase nitric oxide production and further improve endothelial function. Vitamin C supplementation is therefore a V-type method of treating hypertension.

The DRI/RDA of vitamin C is only 90 mg per day in adult males and 75 mg in adult females.[3] Although these doses may prevent scurvy, they are likely too small to yield maximum benefit in reducing blood pressure and cardiovascular disease. Although Linus Pauling himself consumed megadoses of vitamin C, the recommendations of his institute fall shy of these levels, conservatively suggesting an intake of over 400 mg each day. Although many think that very high doses are safe, they may have untoward side effects. In my field there is debate about an association with kidney stones,[92] and I do not recommend supplementation in people with a known history of kidney stones. Daily doses of at least 1000 mg are probably safe,[93] and the DRI/UL is 2000 mg in both adult men and women.[3] As it is difficult to obtain these doses by dietary means, as natural foods are relatively deficient in vitamin C, supplementation of 500 mg a day, which is likely sufficient to obtain most benefits, is suggested. This dose would benefit everyone, with or without hypertension, although there may be an added effect of lowering blood pressure in people with salt-mediated hypertension. Table 5.5 lists several foods with relatively high levels of vitamin C.

Vitamin E

Vitamin E is an important nutrient found in lipid-rich tissue and in cell membranes. Unlike most nutrients, vitamin E is not a single compound but rather a mixture of eight distinct substances. The highest dietary sources are in plant oils such as wheat germ oil, sunflower oil, and safflower oil, which have antioxidant properties and are thought to protect cell membranes from lipid-based free-radical processes. Despite much promise for its role in protecting against heart disease, stroke, and even

Table 5.5 Common Vitamin-C-Rich Foods

Food item	Vitamin C content	Serving size
Orange	70 mg	1 orange, 131 grams
Strawberries	98 mg	1 cup, 166 grams
Kiwi fruit	71 mg	1 medium, 76 grams
Mango	57 mg	1 mango, 207 grams
Cantaloupe	59 mg	1 cup, 160 grams
Papaya	87 mg	1 cup, 140 grams
Orange juice	124 mg	1 cup, 248 grams
Grapefruit juice	94 mg	1 cup, 247 grams
Sweet red peppers	190 mg	1 cup, 149 grams
Sweet green peppers	120 mg	1 cup, 149 grams
Broccoli (cooked)	101 mg	1 cup, 156 grams
Cauliflower (cooked)	55 mg	1 cup, 124 grams
Tomato	23 mg	1 cup, 180 grams

cancer, there is little conclusive data supporting its benefit. Although observational studies suggest a higher intake of vitamin E is associated with a lower risk of heart disease,[94,95] several large randomized studies do not show benefit.[96,97] Its anticipated antioxidant effects on cell membranes would be to minimize the development of atherosclerosis, but evidence for this effect has not yet been realized.[98] In fact, supplementation with high daily doses of over 267 mg (400 IU) may even be associated with greater mortality.[99] As per its effects on blood pressure, the data are also varied, with one study showing reduction with daily supplementation of 133 mg (200 IU),[100] and another showing no effect with 200 mg (300 IU).[101]

The DRI/RDA of vitamin E is only 15 mg (22.5 IU) per day in adult men and women.[3] Given that available data do not clearly show benefit in lowering blood pressure or in protecting from heart disease, it is difficult to suggest further supplementation beyond the daily recommended dose.

Folic acid

Folic acid, also known as vitamin B_9, is an important nutrient with many health effects. Deficient levels can cause anemia and congenital abnormalities such as the neural tube defects spina bifida and anencephaly. Efforts to diminish these ailments, specifically the neural tube defects, have led to folic acid fortification of grain products in many countries. Since 1988, refined cereal grains have been fortified with folic acid in the United States, which has directly reduced folic acid deficiency[102] and, more important, occurrences of neural tube defects.[103] The relationship of folic acid with the amino acid homocysteine has received considerable attention and is an interesting story worth telling, as it involves several well-publicized studies. In the 1960s, an observation that children with homocystinuria, a congenital disease of very elevated homocysteine levels due to inborn errors of metabolism, had premature coronary artery disease. This prompted the hypothesis that homocysteine is a risk factor for heart disease. Since then elevated homocysteine levels in the general public, in most cases only mildly elevated levels, have been considered associated with cardiovascular disease[104,105] and stroke.[106] The mechanism of action is thought to be related to endothelial dysfunction, perhaps mediated by free-radical effects from hydrogen peroxide production.[107] However, there was a lack of consensus that homocysteine was a true risk factor for cardiovascular disease and many thought it was a just a proxy of other ailments, such as kidney disease or inflammation, which were the real risk factors.[108] To answer this question, studies were planned to determine the effects of therapeutic lowering of homocysteine levels on cardiovascular disease. Because folic acid is a cofactor in the enzymatic metabolism of homocysteine, studies utilized its supplementation to lower homocysteine levels and followed its effect on cardiovascular disease. Initial results confirmed the relationship between folic acid supplementation and lower homocysteine levels,[109] although this was already evident as levels across the U.S. population had been reduced since initiation of cereal grain fortification.[110] To the surprise and disappointment of many, several large and credible studies of folic acid supplementation failed to show reduction in cardiovascular events, despite the significantly lowered homocysteine levels.[111–114] There may be some benefit in reducing incidence of stroke.[115] These results have led many physicians to stop recommending folic acid supplementation to their patients. There is also considerable debate about its effect on cancer, both in its *de novo* occurrence and in propagation of established disease.[116] There may be harmful effects from high doses.

Despite these negative findings, several studies have shown a benefit of folic acid supplementation in lowering blood pressure[117–119] and in preventing hypertension.[120] Unfortunately, these studies are few and small, making it difficult to quantify the blood-pressure-lowering effect. In a study of healthy young women, supplementation with 400 μg per day (a relatively small amount) was associated with a decreased risk of developing hypertension.[121] The mechanism of action may involve improved endothelial function[122] due to enhanced vascular nitric oxide production.[123] This effect may be independent of folate-mediated reduction of homocysteine levels.[124] Folic acid supplementation would therefore be a V-type method of lowering blood pressure.

Overall, despite a lack of clear benefit in preventing cardiovascular events, higher dietary folic acid intake may provide benefit in lowering blood pressure and preventing hypertension. A possible concern would

Table 5.6 Common Folic-Acid-Rich Foods

Food item	Folic acid	Serving size
Spinach (cooked or boiled)	263 µg	1 cup, 180 grams
Artichokes (cooked or boiled)	150 µg	1 cup, 168 grams
Broccoli (cooked or boiled)	168 µg	1 cup, 156 grams
Asparagus (cooked or boiled)	89 µg	4 spears, 60 grams
Beets (cooked or boiled)	136 µg	1 cup, 170 grams
Lentils (cooked or boiled)	358 µg	1 cup, 198 grams
Chickpeas (cooked or boiled)	282 µg	1 cup, 164 grams
Split peas (cooked or boiled)	127 µg	1 cup, 196 grams
Pinto beans (cooked or boiled)	294 µg	1 cup, 171 grams
Navy beans (cooked or boiled)	255 µg	1 cup, 182 grams
Kidney beans (cooked or boiled)	230 µg	1 cup, 177 grams
Baker's yeast	164 µg	1 package, 7 grams
Macaroni (enriched and cooked)	167 µg	1 cup, 140 grams
White rice (enriched and cooked)	153 µg	1 cup, 158 grams
Cornmeal (enriched)	476 µg	1 cup, 138 grams
Wheat flour (enriched)	364 µg	1 cup, 125 grams

be the potential for *de novo* occurrence or progression of certain cancers, but this occurs with relatively high doses. Of interest, the bioavailability of supplemental folic acid is almost twice as high as that from natural foods, which means that twice as much must be consumed from natural foods to achieve an effect comparable to supplements. The units of measurement for folic acid are in Dietary Reference Equivalents (DREs), which account for this factor. The DRI/RDA of daily folic acid is 400 µg for adult men and women and 600 µg for pregnant women.[3] Aside from obtaining adequate amounts from food sources, supplementation of 400 µg, a relatively low dose, seems reasonable in people with hypertension. Pregnant women should take prenatal vitamins that often contain higher amounts. Table 5.6 lists several foods with high folic acid content.

Macronutrients

Fiber

Dietary fiber is an important and often neglected part of the diet. The traditional definition of dietary fiber is the indigestible part of plant foods, but more recent additions include analogous synthetic products as well.[125] A typical Western diet includes about 15 grams of fiber per day,[126] compared with about 100 grams in the hunter-gatherer diet of prehistoric times.[4] Its role in promoting healthy bowel movement laxation is commonly known, but there are other beneficial effects as well. Epidemiologic studies suggest that a high-fiber diet is protective against colon and breast cancer.[127] It is also protective of cardiovascular disease,[128] stroke,[129] and the onset of diabetes.[130] These benefits may be due to the association of dietary fiber with improved insulin sensitivity and glucose management[131] and with lower cholesterol levels.[132] However, the story of dietary fiber is considerably more complex, as many subgroups of fiber exist, each with a unique function. Two broad subgroups, the soluble and insoluble fibers, are defined by their ability to dissolve in water and the gut milieu. Most fiber food products contain a mix of these two components but often one type predominates. The insoluble fiber foods are better at promoting bowel movement laxation, whereas the soluble fiber foods are better at protecting from cardiovascular disease and have more benefits in diabetes. The soluble fibers are further divided based on their viscous properties, with higher viscosity associated with added benefit. The U.S. Food and Drug Administration (FDA) has approved two soluble-viscous fibers, psyllium and oat β-glucan fiber, as agents capable of lowering the risk of heart disease.

Dietary fiber has a modest effect on blood pressure. Supplementation with about 11 grams is associated with a decrease in the systolic/diastolic blood pressure of about 1/1 mm Hg.[133] The effect is more pronounced in elderly people and those with hypertension, and can result in as much as a 3/3 mm Hg reduction.[134] Soluble fiber supplements also are more effective than insoluble ones. The mechanism of blood-pressure-lowering is uncertain but may be due to facilitated increases in absorption of nutrients, such as magnesium and potassium, across the intestinal membranes. As the fiber material coats the intestinal walls, it may promote better absorption, which, as previously discussed, is associated with lower blood pressure. Fiber also stimulates secretion of hormones in the intestines, which promotes insulin sensitivity and probably results in better endothelial function. The effect of fiber on blood pressure is very complex and is likely effective in treating both R- and V-types of hypertension.

The DRI/AI for fiber in adults is 14 g for every 1000 calories consumed.[3] This corresponds to 38 g per day in adult males up to 50 years old, 30 g in males over 50 years old, 25 g in adult females up to 50 years old, and 21 g in females over 50 years old. The American Dietetic Association and the American Heart Association both recommend a daily dietary intake of 25 to 30 g of fiber, which all are considerably higher than the typical intake. Table 5.7 lists several high fiber foods and their fiber content.

Dietary fats

The relationship of dietary fats and cholesterol with health is a very important and complex topic. Over the past decades, there have been major shifts in guideline recommendations for optimal dietary intake of fats. At one time, an overall reduction in dietary fat was thought to confer

Table 5.7 Common Fiber-Rich Foods

Food item	Fiber content	Serving size
Raspberries (raw)	8.4 grams	1 cup, 123 grams
Blackberries (raw)	7.6 grams	1 cup, 144 grams
Raisins (raw)	5.8 grams	1 cup, 145 grams
Papaya (raw)	5.5 grams	1 papaya, 304 grams
Pears (raw)	4.4 grams	1 pear, 122 grams
Oranges (raw)	4.3 grams	1 cup, 180 grams
Strawberries (raw)	3.8 grams	1 cup, 166 grams
Apples (raw)	3.7 grams	1 cup, 138 grams
Bananas (raw)	3.6 grams	1 cup, 150 grams
Peas (cooked)	16.3 grams	1 cup, 196 grams
Carrots (cooked)	5.1 grams	1 cup, 156 grams
Cauliflower (cooked)	4.9 grams	1 cup, 180 grams
Potatoes (baked with skin)	4.4 grams	1 potato, 202 grams
Corn (cooked)	3.9 grams	1 cup, 164 grams
Barley (raw)	31.2 grams	1 cup, 200 grams
Bulgar (dry)	25.6 grams	1 cup, 140 grams
Wheat flour (whole grain)	14.6 grams	1 cup, 120 grams
Oat bran (raw)	14.5 grams	1 cup, 94 grams
Lentils (cooked)	15.6 grams	1 cup, 198 grams
Black beans (cooked)	15.0 grams	1 cup, 172 grams
Pinto beans (cooked)	14.7 grams	1 cup, 171 grams
Lima beans (cooked)	13.2 grams	1 cup, 188 grams
Soybeans (cooked)	10.3 grams	1 cup, 172 grams

cardiovascular protection, but later studies did not substantiate this.[135] No doubt the guidelines will undergo further change as more is understood. To adequately appreciate the role of dietary fats in regulating blood pressure and cardiovascular disease, recognition of the individual components and their clinical and mechanistic effects on health need to be understood. Dietary fats are composed of triacylglycerol molecules (i.e., triglycerides), which are formed by the conjugation of a glycerol molecule with three fatty acid molecules (Figure 5.3).

In simple terms, fat is a compound that contains three unique fatty-acid constituents. There are five types of fatty acids of medical importance and their relative composition differs according to food type. They are the trans-fatty acids, saturated fatty acids, monounsaturated fatty acids, omega-6 polyunsaturated fatty acids, and omega-3 polyunsaturated fatty acids. Practically all foods contain a mix of these, but the relative amounts of each can significantly differ. Each fatty acid has a unique effect on cardiovascular disease risk factors, some beneficial and others detrimental.

Fatty acids

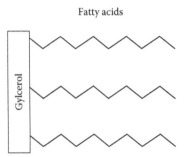

Figure 5.3 The triglyceride structure.

For this reason an overall reduction in dietary fats is not beneficial because the good fats would be reduced along with the bad ones. Much attention is given to the fasting blood lipid profile and its effect on cardiovascular disease. This test measures the blood levels of triglycerides and cholesterol. In humans, lipids are packaged with various proteins into particles called lipoproteins. Of most importance are low-density lipoprotein (LDL), high-density lipoprotein (HDL), and very low-density lipoprotein (VLDL). Each of these contains different proportions of triglycerides, cholesterol, and protein. LDL, also called "bad cholesterol," has high cholesterol content and VLDL has high triglyceride content. Elevated levels of both LDL and total triglycerides, which closely reflect VLDL levels, confer cardiovascular disease risk mostly in the form of atherosclerosis. In contrast, HDL is protective. However, the utility of the fasting blood lipid profile is somewhat limited as the particle sizes of the LDL and HDL also alter cardiovascular risk, and this is not typically measured in the standard test. Smaller LDL particles are associated with increased cardiovascular disease and larger HDL particles (called HDL-2) are protective. The type of dietary fat consumed has significant impact on these lipoprotein levels. Ironically, the amount of cholesterol consumed is less important.[136] Dietary fats also affect the body's systemic inflammatory state by altering levels of anti-inflammatory agents such as nitric oxide and pro-inflammatory agents such as tumor necrosis factor and certain prostaglandins. Together they help regulate overall endothelial function. In summary, the dietary fats have significant effect on lipoprotein levels, the inflammatory state, and endothelial function. As a result, they affect atherosclerosis, blood pressure, and the cardiovascular state.

Trans-fatty acid is the most harmful of the dietary fats. Most of our intake of these fatty acids is from artificial sources as they are produced by chemical alteration of unsaturated fatty acids. Small amounts are consumed from natural products too, as it is present, albeit minimally, in meats and dairy products. Since the introduction of Crisco vegetable shortening in 1902 by the chemist Wilhelm Normann and subsequent marketing of the product, artificial trans fats have been a popular fat alternative. In addition to enhancing the flavor of baked and fried products, this fat has a long shelf life, which makes it desirable to food manufacturers and restaurants. Its consumption significantly increases the risk of developing heart disease, more so than any other fat or food type.[137] It is associated with elevated LDL levels, reduced HDL levels, endothelial dysfunction, inflammation, and atherosclerosis.[138] It is amazing that despite its popularization over the past century, overall life expectancy has increased.

The saturated fats also have harmful cardiovascular effects.[137] Animal products are rich in these fats, as are tropical oils such as palm and coconut oil. They raise LDL levels but have little effect on HDL levels. They also promote endothelial dysfunction, inflammation, and atherosclerosis. In contrast, monounsaturated fats confer protection from cardiovascular disease.[137] The Mediterranean diet, rich in olive oil, is a good source of monounsaturated fats and is very popular for this reason. Although LDL and HDL both are reduced, the ratio of HDL to LDL is improved. These fatty acids also prevent oxidation of LDL particles, an initiating event in atherosclerotic plaque development.

The commonly consumed polyunsaturated fats are divided into omega-3 and omega-6 fatty acids. Omega-3 polyunsaturated fatty acids are found mostly in fish oils and in select plant oils such as canola and flaxseed. The omega-6 polyunsaturated fatty acids are common in other vegetable oils such as sunflower, corn, and soybean. Despite favorably altering the lipoprotein levels, there is a suggestion that the omega-6 polyunsaturated fats are associated with cardiovascular disease. This may be due to its conversion to arachidonic acid, which is a pro-inflammatory substance. There is also increased potential in forming oxidized LDL particles. Both of these processes may cause atherosclerosis and endothelial dysfunction. However, compared with the saturated fats and trans fats, omega-6 polyunsaturated fats are likely protective of cardiovascular disease, although not by as much as the monounsaturated fats.[139-141] The omega-3 polyunsaturated fats have received much positive attention for their ability to protect from cardiovascular disease. Interest began with the observation that Greenland Eskimos who consume large amounts of this fat rarely develop heart disease.[142] In the years since this discovery, several large studies have shown significant cardiovascular benefit from consumption of omega-3 polyunsaturated fats.[143,144] The main dietary sources of these fats are fatty fish—especially salmon, herring, sardines, and tuna—and plant products such as canola oil, flaxseed oil, and walnuts. However, the fatty acids from fish are eicosapentaenoic acid (EPA) and docosahexaenoic acid (DHA) and from plants is alpha-linolenic acid (ALA). EPA and DHA are more direct inhibitors of inflammation but ALA must first be converted into EPA and DHA to be effective. The conversion rate for this process is quite variable but a reasonable estimate would be only about 10%.[145] This means that 10 times the amount of plant-derived ALA needs to be consumed to equal the potency of fish-derived EPA or DHA. The mechanisms by which omega-3 polyunsaturated fats protect from cardiovascular disease are different from other fatty acids. There is a minimal effect on the overall LDL and HDL levels, although the particle size of both is increased, which has a beneficial effect. The blood triglyceride level is also significantly lowered.[146] Much of the cardiovascular protection comes from prevention of cardiac arrhythmias and sudden death events.[147] Endothelial function is also improved as nitric oxide production is increased[148] and pro-inflammatory mediators are decreased.[149] Among all the fatty acid types, substitution and addition of omega-3 polyunsaturated fats seems the best way to prevent cardiovascular disease.

Dietary fats also affect the blood pressure, and the different types of fats have different effects. The omega-3 polyunsaturated fats appear to be the most potent in reducing blood pressure. As previously described, the three main types of dietary omega-3 polyunsaturated fats are the fish oils EPA and DHA and the plant oil ALA. Because ALA must be converted to EPA and DHA to become active, most studies have focused on the fish oils. A typical response to fish oil supplementation in people with hypertension is reduction in systolic/diastolic blood pressure of 3.4–5.5/2.0–3.5 mm Hg.[150–152] In people with normal blood pressure, a more modest reduction of about 1/1 mm Hg is observed. Older people also tend to have a better response. Although there is debate about the amount of omega-3 polyunsaturated fat needed to fully achieve this effect, it appears that a modest intake of 500 to 1000 mg of fish-derived omega-3 polyunsaturated fat per day or 3500 to 7000 mg per week is sufficient.[153] This can be accomplished with one serving of fatty fish such as salmon or tuna several times a week. Commercially available fish oil supplements in either pill or oil form are also available. In the United States, Lovaza® is a prescribed medication and each 1 g capsule contains about 840 mg of omega-3 polyunsaturated fats. The over-the-counter fish oil capsules often contain less, with between 200 and 800 mg of omega-3 polyunsaturated fats in each 1 g capsule. The side effects from such doses are minimal. Plant-derived omega-3 polyunsaturated fat, specifically ALA, should have similar effects to the fish oils although much higher doses would be needed. The mechanism by which blood pressure is lowered is similar to those discussed for cardiovascular benefits. Endothelial function is improved by reduction of pro-inflammatory mediators and enhanced nitric oxide production. Endovascular and red blood cell wall membrane fluidity is also improved by an alteration of the cholesterol and phospholipid composition of the cell wall,[154,155] thus improving the fluidity of blood within the vascular system and to subsequent lowering of blood pressure. Consumption of omega-3 polyunsaturated fat would therefore be a V-type method of treating hypertension. Monounsaturated fats, which are abundant in the Mediterranean diet rich in olive oil, also are associated with lowering blood pressure.[156,157] Omega-6 polyunsaturated fats may be associated with a lower blood pressure,[158] although the evidence is less clear. In contrast, saturated fats are associated with increased blood pressure.[158] Table 5.8 summarizes the effects of the various dietary fats.

Table 5.8 Cardiovascular Effects of Dietary Fats

Omega-3 polyunsaturated fats

Lower blood pressure
Lower triglycerides
Minimal effect on LDL and HDL
Protective of cardiovascular disease
Reduce cardiac arrhythmias
Prevent atherosclerosis
Improve endothelial function

Monounsaturated fats

Lower blood pressure
Lower LDL and HDL
Increase HDL:LDL (ratio)
Protective of cardiovascular disease
Prevent atherosclerosis
Improve endothelial function

Omega-6 polyunsaturated fats

Likely lower blood pressure
Likely are protective of cardiovascular disease

Saturated fats

Raise blood pressure
Increase LDL
Mediate cardiovascular disease
Cause endothelial dysfunction
Cause systemic inflammation
Cause atherosclerosis

Trans fats

Raise blood pressure
Increase LDL and decrease HDL
Mediate cardiovascular disease
Cause endothelial dysfunction
Cause systemic inflammation
Cause atherosclerosis

The Dietary Guidelines for Americans suggest a total fat intake of 20% to 35% of total daily calories.[1] Of these, less than 10% should be from saturated fats, and trans fats should be restricted entirely. Monounsaturated fats, plant-derived omega-6 and omega-3 polyunsaturated fats, and fish-derived omega-3 fats should make up the remaining fat calories. Total daily cholesterol intake should be limited to 300 mg. In adults with risk factors for cardiovascular disease, less than 7% of total daily calories should be from saturated fats and total daily cholesterol intake should be limited to 200 mg. The NCEP expert panel recommends similar values.[2] They suggest a total fat intake of up to 35% of daily calories, but break down the fat types to include less than 7% from saturated fats, up to 10% from polyunsaturated fats, and up to 20% from monounsaturated fats. Cholesterol intake should be less than 200 mg each day. No specific recommendations are provided for omega-3 polyunsaturated fats, but the DRI/AI of ALA is 1.6 g per day for adult males and 1.1 g for adult females. As previously discussed, plant-derived ALA is considerably less efficacious than the fish-derived fats. Daily consumption of 500 to 1000 mg of fish-derived omega-3 polyunsaturated fat is probably sufficient to obtain most of the cardiovascular and blood-pressure-lowering benefits. On a weekly basis, 3500 to 7000 mg would be needed. This can be achieved with a steady diet of fatty fish several times a week or with a daily supplement of 1 g of Lovaza or 2 g of over-the-counter fish oil. Comparable intake of plant-derived omega-3 polyunsaturated fat (i.e., ALA) would be more difficult because at least 5 to 10 g would be needed and even this may not be enough for significant benefit. Table 5.9 lists several rich sources of omega-3 polyunsaturated fats.

Carbohydrates

Carbohydrates are made from building blocks of sugar molecules and comprise the majority of the calories of most diets. They are classified as either simple sugars (e.g., monosaccharides and disaccharides) or as complex carbohydrates (e.g., starches or polysaccharides). The monosaccharides are individual sugar molecules such as glucose or fructose (Figure 5.4), and disaccharides are two-sugar molecules chemically conjugated, such as sucrose, which contains one glucose and one fructose molecule (Figure 5.4). The complex carbohydrates contain many sugar molecules. Dietary fiber is technically a carbohydrate, but in humans it is not digested to individual sugar molecules and therefore should be excluded in the dietary carbohydrate count. However, dietary fiber is often included in the total carbohydrate count on the nutrient source labels of many food products, which may be a source of confusion. Although a number of popular diets recommend a relatively low carbohydrate intake, the major guidelines still suggest carbohydrates should comprise about

Table 5.9 Common Omega-3-Rich Foods

Food item	Omega-3 content	Serving size
Salmon (farmed)	4504 mg	6.0 ounces
Salmon (wild)	1774 mg	6.0 ounces
Herring (Atlantic)	1712 mg	3.0 ounces
Golden bass	1358 mg	5.3 ounces
Anchovy	1165 mg	2.0 ounces
Mackerel (Atlantic)	1059 mg	3.1 ounces
Swordfish	868 mg	3.7 ounces
Tuna (white albacore)	733 mg	3.0 ounces
Mussels	665 mg	3.0 ounces
Oysters	585 mg	3.0 ounces
Trout	581 mg	2.2 ounces
Sardines	556 mg	2.0 ounces
Flaxseeds	2200 mg	1.0 Tbsp
Canola oil	1300 mg	1.0 Tbsp
Flaxseed oil	8500 mg	1.0 Tbsp
Walnuts	700 mg	1.0 Tbsp

Source: Data for fish sources from Mozaffarian D, Rimm EB, Fish intake, contaminants, and human health: Evaluating the risks and the benefits, *JAMA*, 2006;296:1885–1899.

50% of caloric intake. Of course, the guidelines advocate fruits and vegetables as the primary sources, which unfortunately have become unpopular in Western diets in favor of fast foods and refined carbohydrates. Over the past century, simple sugars have been replacing dietary fiber in Western diets.[159] This is especially true in the United States, where—largely fueled by the farming industry—high fructose corn syrup (HFCS) has become popular and is now the most commonly used sweetener. Unfortunately, many health problems have been associated with this shift in carbohydrate use. Although there is continued debate over the potentially harmful effects of a high-carbohydrate diet, the effects of elevated blood glucose levels are clearly detrimental. A useful tool in estimating the glycemic

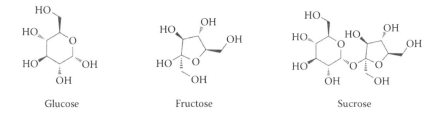

Glucose   Fructose   Sucrose

Figure 5.4 Simple sugars.

impact of foods is the glycemic index, which measures the increases in blood glucose levels in response to various foods over a 2-hour period. The values are compared to the response of a 50 g meal of either white bread or pure glucose. For example, using white bread as the standard, a 50 g meal would equate to a 100% value. A 50 g carbohydrate meal of an apple has a glycemic index of only 55(%) as it causes a smaller rise in the 2-hour glucose level. This suggests that the blood glucose effect of these two carbohydrate sources are very different, as the white bread causes an immediate rise, whereas the apple has a slower and more sustained effect on blood glucose. Generally, low-glycemic-index foods are considered healthier. Although the glycemic index has become a useful marker, there are many factors that can significantly alter these values, and it should be used with caution. The degree of ripeness of a fruit, for example, can affect its glycemic index as well as the intake of other nutrients as in meals containing a mix of fats, proteins, and vitamins. These factors affect the body's ability to digest and absorb this nutrient. Nonetheless, it is a reasonably consistent gauge with which to compare the effect of various foods on blood glucose levels.[160] Another useful measure, the glycemic load, is simply the product of the glycemic index of a food multiplied by a typical portion size. As an example, if a typical apple contains 21 g of carbohydrates, the glycemic load would be 12 g per serving (21 g × 55% = 12 g). Because the glycemic load deals with typical serving sizes, it is a more convenient measure.

Pure glucose is rapidly absorbed as it requires no further enzymatic breakdown, and therefore has a very high glycemic index. Fructose has a glycemic index of only 19 and causes just a minimal rise in blood glucose levels within the 2-hour period following ingestion. This is due to its slow conversion to glucose and some effects on glucose absorption. However, despite its low glycemic index, fructose has many detrimental health effects. HFCS typically is composed of about equal portions of glucose and fructose, and has a glycemic index of 55 to 60. The type of complex carbohydrate also has a significant impact on the glycemic index of the food. There are two types of complex carbohydrates: amylose and amylopectin. Amylose is a large linear chain typically containing 300 to 600 sugar molecules, whereas amylopectin is a branched structure containing up to 6000 sugar molecules. These structural differences are important as they alter the food's potential to raise blood glucose levels. The linear array of the amylose starches can be viewed as a ball of string tightly wrapped around itself (Figure 5.5). When this ball reaches the stomach and small intestine, most of the sugar molecules are insulated within the structure protected from enzymatic breakdown. Amylopectin can be viewed as a cluster of grapes (Figure 5.5), which would make it easy for the gastrointestinal enzymes to pluck off the sugar molecules. Therefore,

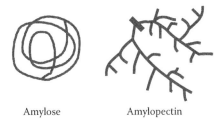

Amylose   Amylopectin

Figure 5.5 Complex carbohydrates. (Courtesy of Shani Strenger from Shilo, Israel.)

foods with high amylose starch content have a lower glycemic index than those with more amylopectin. Of course, most foods contain many types of carbohydrate and it is the varied mix of simple sugars, amylose, and amylopectin that contribute to the glycemic index.

The theory behind the adverse health effects of elevated glucose levels is quite complex but convincing.[161] Unfortunately, large conclusive studies are not available as it would be unethical to subject people to unhealthy diets for a study. Most of the clinical data comes from observational studies in humans and experimental studies in animals, which, although reasonably suggestive, do not provide absolute proof. Diets containing high glycemic-index foods cause a rapid increase in blood glucose levels. In the immediate period, typically within the first 2 hours, a counterregulatory response occurs resulting in increased insulin and decreased glucagon secretion from the pancreas (Figure 5.6). Liver production of glucose is also diminished and muscle uptake is increased to buffer the high blood-glucose levels. However, this response is often too robust, and within 2 to 4 hours after the meal the intended effect is surpassed causing blood glucose levels to drop too far. This causes another counterregulatory

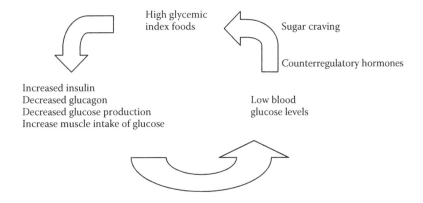

High glycemic
index foods

Sugar craving

Counterregulatory hormones

Increased insulin
Decreased glucagon
Decreased glucose production
Increase muscle intake of glucose

Low blood
glucose levels

Figure 5.6 Effect of high-glycemic foods on glucose metabolism.

response with release of pro-glucose hormones and subsequent increase in blood glucose levels (Figure 5.6). The craving for sugars often perpetuates the cycle as people again consume high-glycemic-index foods. Within 4 to 6 hours after the meal, blood glucose levels are restored or somewhat increased and triglyceride levels also may become elevated. Low-glycemic meals avoid this seesaw effect by more slowly and steadily increasing blood glucose levels. Such meals also provide more satiety and a higher resting energy expenditure (i.e., higher basal metabolic rate), both of which promote weight loss and are protective of cardiovascular disease.[162] Animal studies comparing high- and low-glycemic diets of equal caloric intake show higher body fat and lower muscle mass in the high-glycemic group.[163] Other untoward effects of high-glycemic meals include increased insulin resistance in the muscle and liver due to higher insulin and triglyceride levels. Pancreatic β-cell failure may also occur, leading to diminished insulin output and potentially to diabetes in susceptible individuals. Several large observational studies have found an association between high-glycemic and low-fiber diets with the development of diabetes,[164,165] although others have not.[166] High-glycemic diets also are associated with altered cholesterol levels,[167] increased systemic inflammation,[168] and endothelial dysfunction.[169] Studies also suggest an association with coronary heart disease,[170,171] and possible links to increased rates of colorectal[172] and pancreatic cancer.[173]

Special attention must be given to the relatively recent increases in consumption of large amounts of fructose, mostly in the form of HFCS. This is particularly important in the United States, where it is commonly used as a sweetener. Unlike table sugar that is a solid, HFCS is a liquid that makes it easily transported and readily miscible in food products. Its caloric value and glycemic index are comparable to table sugar. As previously mentioned, HFCS has about equal parts of the simple unattached sugars glucose and fructose. Because of biochemical nuances in its metabolism, fructose bypasses many of the regulatory steps of glucose metabolism and, when consumed in large amounts, causes increased weight gain, fat storage, increased insulin resistance, elevated triglyceride levels, and hypertension.[174] HFCS clearly is a health hazard especially as it has largely supplanted the intake of dietary fiber.

The effect of carbohydrates on blood pressure is not clear, as surprisingly few large and conclusive studies have been performed. One technical limitation for such trials is that dietary sources of carbohydrates are quite varied, making it difficult to draw general conclusions about this class of macronutrient. For example, a high-carbohydrate diet may contain healthy, relatively low-glycemic load foods such as fruits and vegetables but also may contain refined carbohydrates and simple sugars such as white-flour products and sweets. Despite having comparable amounts of carbohydrate, the healthy diet is more likely to result in better cardiovascular effects and lower blood pressure. Of the large studies that have addressed this issue, several have shown benefit of a low-carbohydrate diet in lowering blood pressure,[175,176] whereas others have not.[177,178] Most of these studies do not provide any details about the type of carbohydrate consumed nor do they focus on people with hypertension. However, the OmniHeart study is unique,[175] as it includes only people with hypertension and prehypertension, and compares diets that are consistent with the healthy standards of the Dietary Guidelines for Americans. Specifically, the study compares diets with 10% differences in carbohydrates, fats, and proteins, and concludes that reduced carbohydrate intake is associated with a modest reduction in blood pressure. In the hypertensive group there was a reduction of 3/2 mm Hg and a reduction in the prehypertensive group of 1/0–1 mm Hg. An understanding of the mechanisms by which carbohydrates regulate blood pressure may be helpful in explaining the discrepancies between these studies. Blood glucose and insulin levels importantly and uniquely affect the blood pressure. Blood glucose levels, especially following a sudden elevation (i.e., glucose excursion) cause vasoconstriction[179] with a subsequent rise in blood pressure. This effect is mediated through endothelial dysfunction.[169] Nitric oxide levels are diminished and vasoconstricting mediators such as endothelin-1 are increased. The effect of elevated insulin levels on the vasculature appears to be opposite that of glucose as it initially dilates the vessels and lowers the blood pressure.[180] However, there is an immediate sympathetic response to this lowered blood pressure resulting in vasoconstriction and a near restoration of the blood pressure. When consuming a carbohydrate meal, the initial glucose excursion and subsequent insulin release both contribute to changes in the blood pressure. In healthy people with normal endothelial function, these two effects roughly counterbalance each other and result in only a small effect on the blood pressure. However, in people with endothelial dysfunction, such as those with hypertension or diabetes, the sympathetic counterresponse to insulin causes an exaggerated constricting effect that overwhelms the initial blood-pressure-lowering effect. In these people, both the glucose excursion and the insulin response cause constriction of the vessels with a subsequent rise in blood pressure. This may explain the larger effect of carbohydrates in the hypertensive group of the OmniHeart study.

A low carbohydrate diet would be a V-type method of lowering blood pressure. The Dietary Guidelines for Americans suggests a total carbohydrate intake of 45% to 65% of total daily calories.[1] The NCEP expert panel recommends similar values.[2] Of course, these guidelines suggest carbohydrate intake from healthy and relatively low-glycemic-index sources such as fruits, vegetables, and whole grains. This type of carbohydrate also contains important minerals, vitamins, and antioxidants, which are relatively scarce in processed carbohydrates such as cake, sweets, and white

Table 5.10 Common Low-Glycemic-Index Foods

Food item	Glycemic index	Glycemic load (serving size)
Cherries	22	3 (120 grams)
Grapefruit	25	3 (120 grams)
Apple	38	6 (180 grams)
Orange	43	5 (120 grams)
Grapes	46	8 (120 grams)
Banana	52	12 (120 grams)
Tomato juice	38	4 (250 ml)
Carrot juice	43	14 (250 ml)
Apple juice	44	13 (250 ml)
Peanuts	14	1 (50 grams)
Cashews	22	3 (50 grams)
Yam	37	13 (150 grams)
Carrots	47	3 (80 grams)
Green peas	48	3 (80 grams)
Barley (pearled)	25	11 (150 grams)
Long-grain rice (white)	56	24 (150 grams)
Chickpeas (boiled)	28	8 (150 grams)
Kidney beans	28	7 (150 grams)
Lentils	29	5 (150 grams)
Lima beans	32	10 (150 grams)
Milk (whole)	27	3 (250 ml)
Milk (skim)	32	4 (250 ml)
Yogurt	36	3 (200 grams)
Bread (rye, pumpernickel)	41	5 (30 grams)
Bread (stone-ground whole wheat)	59	7 (30 grams)
Fettuccini (egg)	40	18 (180 grams)
Spaghetti (white)	38	18 (180 grams)

Source: Data for glycemic index compared with glucose load from: Foster-Powell K, Holt SH, Brand-Miller JC, International table of glycemic index and glycemic load values, *Am J Clin Nutr,* 2002;76:5–56.

bread. In treating hypertension, it may be beneficial to try to keep to the lower level of 45% of total calories. Table 5.10 lists common foods with low glycemic indexes.

Protein

Protein makes up the remainder of dietary calories, typically contributing the least. Proteins are comprised of amino acid molecules, of which humans and other animals utilize about 20 different types. At one time, high-protein diets were considered harmful to health and proper blood pressure regulation, however, this notion has been mostly discredited. This supposition was partly based on anecdotal evidence from studies promoting the beneficial health effects of vegetarian diets, which are typically low in protein content.[181,182] Because the coincidental intake of nutrients and antioxidants of a vegetarian diet certainly contribute to its healthful effects, these conclusions are now in doubt. In fact, large credible studies such as the Nurses' Health Study suggest a protective cardiovascular effect from a high-protein diet,[183] although plant-derived proteins may be more beneficial than animal proteins.[184] High-protein diets also may decrease the risk of hemorrhagic stroke.[185] Despite these seemingly beneficial effects, high-protein diets are associated with progression of kidney disease, especially in individuals with impaired renal function.[186]

Although some epidemiologic studies suggest an association between dietary protein consumption and elevated blood pressure,[22] most show the opposite trend and an overall lowering effect on blood pressure is well accepted. Some of these studies show a lowering effect from nonspecific sources of protein,[176,187] whereas others note this effect only from plant-derived protein.[178,188] The various components of animal and plant protein may contribute to these findings as animal protein contains nutrients such as saturated fats, which themselves cause blood pressure increases; whereas vegetable protein has healthful minerals, vitamins, and antioxidants that lower blood pressure. The OmniHeart study probably provides the clearest evidence of the role of proteins in regulating blood pressure as it compares dietary protein with other macronutrient intake in a balanced diet of adequate minerals and vitamins.[175] The protein contribution is also well balanced with a mix of vegetable, lean meats, and poultry sources. With a 10% increase in caloric intake from carbohydrates to proteins, a modest lowering in blood pressure is observed. In this study, people with hypertension experienced a decrease of 3/2 mm Hg and those with prehypertension showed a decrease of 1/1 mm Hg. There was no difference between the increased protein and increased fat groups. Therefore, high-protein diets appear to reduce blood pressure, although there is probably an added benefit from plant-derived over animal-derived protein.

An interesting class of compounds called flavonoids may contribute to the favorable effect of vegetable protein. These are water-soluble plant pigments commonly found in foods such as onions, cocoa, tea, apples, citrus fruits, berries, and soy.[189] Soy protein causes a small reduction in blood pressure and may also improve serum lipid levels.[190] Because protein is made of a mixture of 20 types of amino acids, the precise cause in lowering blood pressure is complex. Each amino acid confers unique effect, some with blood-pressure-lowering properties and others not. Glutamic acid, perhaps the most common amino acid constituent of protein—particularly vegetable protein—is directly associated with lower blood pressure.[191] Its effect arises mostly from improved endothelial function due to antioxidant properties and increased nitric oxide production. Proline, phenylalanine, and serine are also relatively common vegetable protein amino acids that are associated with lower blood pressure.[191] Arginine, as the substrate for the enzyme nitric oxide synthase and a direct production of nitric oxide, also can lower blood pressure.[192] Tyrosine[193] and tryptophan[194] may lower blood pressure by decreasing central sympathetic nervous system activity. Dietary protein is comprised of so many independent sources, thus it is difficult to ascribe a single mechanism to its ability to lower blood pressure, although there is a strong V-type contribution.

The Dietary Guidelines for Americans suggests a total daily protein intake of 10% to 35% of total daily calories.[1] In treating hypertension, it may be beneficial to target the upper side of this range and to focus on plant protein sources.

References

1. U.S. Department of Agriculture and U.S. Department of Health and Human Services. *Dietary Guidelines for Americans, 2010.* 7th ed. Washington, DC: U.S. Government Printing Office; December 2010. www.health.gov/dietary-guidelines/dga2010/DietaryGuidelines2010.pdf.
2. National Cholesterol Education Program (NCEP) Expert Panel on Detection, Evaluation, and Treatment of High Blood Cholesterol in Adults (Adult Treatment Panel III). Third report of the National Cholesterol Education Program (NCEP) Expert Panel on Detection, Evaluation, and Treatment of High Blood Cholesterol in Adults (Adult Treatment Panel III) final report. *Circulation.* 2002;106:3143–3421.
3. Otten JJ, Hellwig JP, Meyers LD. *Dietary DRI Reference Intakes: The Essential Guide to Nutrient Requirements.* Washington, DC: The National Academies Press; 2006.
4. Eaton SB, Eaton SB 3rd, Konner MJ. Paleolithic nutrition revisited: A twelve-year retrospective on its nature and implications. *Eur J Clin Nutr.* 1997;51:207–216.
5. Engstrom A, Tobelmann RC, Albertson AM. Sodium intake trends and food choices. *Am J Clin Nutr.* 1997;65(suppl):704S–707S.
6. Oliver W, Cohen EL, Neel JV. Blood pressure, sodium intake and sodium related hormones in the Yanomamo Indians, a "no-salt" culture. *Circulation.* 1975;52:146–151.
7. Poulter NR, Khaw KT, Hopwood BE, et al. The Kenyan Luo migration study: Observations on the initiation of a rise in blood pressure. *BMJ.* 1990;300:967–972.
8. Kaplan NM. Dietary salt intake and blood pressure. *JAMA.* 1984;251:1429–1430.
9. Hofman A, Hazebroek A, Valkenburg HA. A randomized trial of sodium intake and blood pressure in newborn infants. *JAMA.* 1983;250:370–373.
10. Geleijnse JM, Hofman A, Witteman JC, Hazebroek AA, Valkenburg HA, Grobbee DE. Long-term effects of neonatal sodium restriction on blood pressure. *Hypertension.* 1997;29:913–917.

11. Intersalt Cooperative Research Group. Intersalt: An international study of electrolyte excretion and blood pressure. Results for 24-hour urinary sodium and potassium excretion. *BMJ.* 1988;297:319–328.

12. Midgley JP, Matthew AG, Greenwood CM, Logan AG. Effects of reduced dietary sodium on blood pressure: A meta-analysis of randomized controlled trials. *JAMA.* 1996;275:1590–1597.

13. Graudal NA, Galløe AM, Garred P. Effects of sodium, restriction on blood pressure, renin, aldosterone, catecholamines, cholesterols, and triglyceride: A meta-analysis. *JAMA.* 1998;279:1383–1391.

14. Cutler JA, Follmann D, Allender PS. Randomized trials of sodium reduction: An overview. *Am J Clin Nutr.* 1997;65(suppl):643S–651S.

15. Law MR. Epidemiologic evidence on salt and blood pressure. *Am J Hypertens.* 1997;10:42S–45S.

16. Messerli FH, Schmieder RE, Weir MR. Salt. A perpetrator of hypertensive target organ disease? *Arch Intern Med.* 1997;157:2449–2452.

17. Sakhaee K, Harvey JA, Padalino PK, Whitson P, Pak CY. The potential role of salt abuse on the risk for kidney stone formation. *J Urol.* 1993;150:310–312.

18. Alderman MH, Madhavan S, Cohen H, Sealey JE, Laragh JH. Low urinary sodium is associated with greater risk of myocardial infarction among treated hypertensive men. *Hypertension.* 1995;25:1144–1152.

19. Alderman MH, Cohen H, Madhavan S. Dietary sodium intake and mortality: The National Health and Nutrition Examination Survey (NHANES I). *Lancet.* 1998;351:781–785.

20. He FJ, Markandu ND, Sagnella GA, MacGregor GA. Importance of the renin system in determining blood pressure fall with salt restriction in black and white hypertensives. *Hypertension.* 1998;32:820–824.

21. Alderman MH. Salt, blood pressure and health: A cautionary tale. *Int J Epidemiol.* 2002;31:311–315.

22. Hajjar IM, Grim CE, George V, Kotchen TA. Impact of diet on blood pressure and age-related changes in blood pressure in the U.S. population: Analysis of NHANES III. *Arch Intern Med.* 2001;161:589–593.

23. Langford HG. Dietary potassium and hypertension: Epidemiologic data. *Ann Intern Med.* 1983;98(5 Pt 2):770–772.

24. Veterans Administration Cooperative Study Group on Antihypertensive Agents. Urinary and serum electrolytes in untreated black and white hypertensives. *J Chronic Dis.* 1987;40:839–847.

25. Kawano Y, Minami J, Takishita S, Omae T. Effects of potassium supplementation on office, home, and 24-hour blood pressure in patients with essential hypertension. *Am J Hypertens.* 1998;11:1141–1146.

26. Whelton PK, He J, Cutler JA, et al. Effects of oral potassium on blood pressure: Meta-analysis of randomized controlled clinical trials. *JAMA.* 1997;277:1624–1632.

27. MacGregor GA, Smith SJ, Markandu ND, Banks RA, Sagnella GA. Moderate potassium supplementation in essential hypertension. *Lancet.* 1982;2(8298):567–570.

28. Bazzano LA, He J, Ogden LG, et al. Dietary potassium intake and risk of stroke in U.S. men and women: National Health and Nutrition Examination Survey I epidemiologic follow-up study. *Stroke.* 2001;32:1473–1480.

29. Khaw KT, Barrett-Connor E. Dietary potassium and stroke-associated mortality: A 12-year prospective population study. *N Engl J Med.* 1987;316:235–240.

30. Tobian L. The Volhard lecture. Potassium and sodium in hypertension. *J Hypertens Suppl.* 1988;6:S12–S24.
31. Brunner HR, Baer L, Sealey JE, Ledingham JG, Laragh JH. The influence of potassium administration and of potassium deprivation on plasma renin in normal and hypertensive subjects. *J Clin Invest.* 1970;49:2128–2138.
32. Tannen R. Effects of potassium on blood pressure control. *Ann Intern Med.* 1983;98(5 Pt 2):773–780.
33. van Mierlo LA, Arends LR, Streppel MT, et al. Blood pressure response to calcium supplementation: A meta-analysis of randomized controlled trials. *J Hum Hypertens.* 2006;20:571–580.
34. Allender PS, Cutler JA, Follmann D, Cappuccio FP, Pryer J, Elliott P. Dietary calcium and blood pressure: A meta-analysis of randomized clinical trials. *Ann Intern Med.* 1996;124:825–831.
35. Davies KM, Heaney RP, Recker RR. Calcium intake and body weight. *J Clin Endocrinol Metab.* 2000;85:4635–4638.
36. Jorde R, Sundsfjord J, Haug E, Bonaa KH. Relation between low calcium intake, parathyroid hormone, and blood pressure. *Hypertension.* 2000;35:1154–1159.
37. Gennari C, Heaney RP, Recker RR, et al. Hypertension and primary hyperparathyroidism: The role of adrenergic and renin–angiotensin–aldosterone systems. *Miner Electrolyte Metab.* 1995;21:77–81.
38. Appel LJ, Moore TJ, Obarzanek E, et al. A clinical trial of the effects of dietary patterns on blood pressure. *N Engl J Med.* 1997;336:1117–1124.
39. Beierwaltes WH. The role of calcium in the regulation of renin secretion. *Am J Physiol Renal Physiol.* 2010;298: F1–F11.
40. Klar J, Sigl M, Obermayer B, Schweda F, Krämer BK, Kurtz A. Calcium inhibits renin gene expression by transcriptional and posttranscriptional mechanisms. *Hypertension.* 2005;46:1340–1346.
41. Karppanen H, Karppanen P, Mervaala E. Why and how to implement sodium, potassium, calcium, and magnesium changes in food items and diets? *J Hum Hypertens.* 2005;19:S10–S19.
42. Mizushima S, Cappuccio FP, Nichols R, Elliott P. Dietary magnesium intake and blood pressure: A qualitative overview of the observational studies. *J Hum Hypertens.* 1998;12:447–453.
43. Jee SH, Miller ER 3rd, Guallar E, Singh VK, Appel LJ, Klag MJ. The effect of magnesium supplementation on blood pressure: A meta-analysis of randomized clinical trials. *Am J Hypertens.* 2002;15:691–696.
44. Kawano Y, Matsuoka H, Takishita S, Omae T. Effects of magnesium supplementation in hypertensive patients: Assessment by office, home, and ambulatory blood pressures. *Hypertension.* 1998;32:260–265.
45. Dyckner T, Wester PO. Effect of magnesium on blood pressure. *Br Med J (Clin Res Ed).* 1983;286:1847–1849.
46. Zhang A, Cheng TP, Altura BM. Magnesium regulates intracellular free ionized calcium concentration and cell geometry in vascular smooth muscle cells. *Biochim Biophys Acta.* 1992;1134:25–29.
47. Shimosawa T, Takano K, Ando K, Fujita T. Magnesium inhibits norepinephrine release by blocking N-type calcium channels at peripheral sympathetic nerve endings. *Hypertension.* 2004;44:897–902.
48. Whang R, Whang DD, Ryan MP. Refractory potassium repletion. A consequence of magnesium deficiency. *Arch Intern Med.* 1992;152:40–45.

49. Kendrick J, Targher G, Smits G, Chonchol M. 25-hydroxyvitamin D deficiency is independently associated with cardiovascular disease in the Third National Health and Nutrition Examination Survey. *Atherosclerosis.* 2009;205:255–260.

50. Giovannucci E, Liu Y, Hollis BW, Rimm EB. 25-hydroxyvitamin D and risk of myocardial infarction in men: A prospective study. *Arch Intern Med.* 2008;168:1174–1180.

51. Wang T, Pencina MJ, Booth SL, et al. Vitamin D deficiency and risk of cardiovascular disease. *Circulation.* 2008;117:503–511.

52. Poole KE, Loveridge N, Barker PJ, et al. Reduced vitamin D in acute stroke. *Stroke.* 2006;37:243–245.

53. Melamed ML, Michos ED, Post W, Astor B. 25-hydrox vitamin D levels and the risk of mortality in the general population. *Arch Intern Med.* 2008;168:1629–1637.

54. Chiu KC, Chu A, Go VL, Saad MF. Hypovitaminosis D is associated with insulin resistance and β cell dysfunction. *Am J Clin Nutr.* 2004;79:820–825.

55. Martins D, Wolf M, Pan D, et al. Prevalence of cardiovascular risk factors and the serum levels of 25-hydroxyvitamin D in the United States; data from the Third National Health and Nutrition Examination Survey. *Arch Intern Med.* 2007;167:1159–1165.

56. Hagström E, Hellman P, Larsson TE, et al. Plasma parathyroid hormone and the risk of cardiovascular mortality in the community. *Circulation.* 2009;119:2765–2771.

57. Bhuriya R, Li S, Chen SC, McCullough PA, Bakris GL. Plasma parathyroid hormone level and prevalent cardiovascular disease in CKD stages 3 and 4: An analysis from the Kidney Early Evaluation Program (KEEP). *Am J Kidney Dis.* 2009;53:S3-S10.

58. Chiu KC, Chuang LM, Lee NP, et al. Insulin sensitivity is inversely correlated with plasma intact parathyroid hormone level. *Metabolism.* 2000;49:1501–1505.

59. Reis JP, von Mühlen D, Miller ER 3rd. Relation of 25-hydroxyvitamin D and parathyroid hormone levels with metabolic syndrome among U.S. adults. *Eur J Endocrinol.* 2008;159:41–48.

60. Judd SE, Nanes MS, Ziegler TR, Wilson PW, Tangpricha V. Optimal vitamin D status attenuates the age-associated increase in systolic blood pressure in white Americans; results from the Third National Health and Nutrition Examination Survey. *Am J Clin Nutr.* 2008;87:136–141.

61. Kristal-Boneh E, Froom P, Harari G, Ribak J. Association of calcitriol and blood pressure in normotensive men. *Hypertension.* 1997;30:1289–1294.

62. Scragg R, Sowers M, Bell C. Serum 25-hydroxyvitamin D, ethnicity, and blood pressure in the Third National Health and Nutrition Examination Survey. *Am J Hypertens.* 2007;20:713–719.

63. Rostand SG. Ultraviolet light may contribute to geographic and racial blood pressure differences. *Hypertension.* 1997;30(2 Pt 1):150–156.

64. Forman JP, Giovannucci E, Holmes MD, et al. Plasma 25-hydroxyvitamin D levels and risk of incident hypertension. *Hypertension.* 2007;49:1063–1069.

65. Snijder MB, Lips P, Seidell JC, et al. Vitamin D status and parathyroid hormone levels in relation to blood pressure: A population-based study in older men and women. *J Intern Med.* 2007;261:558–565.

66. Jorde R, Bonaa KH, Sundsfjord J. Population based study on serum ionized calcium, serum parathyroid hormone, and blood pressure: The Tromsø study. *Eur J Endocrinol.* 1999;141:350–357.

67. Jorde R, Svartberg J, Sundsfjord J. Serum parathyroid hormone as a predictor of increase in systolic blood pressure in men. *J Hypertens.* 2005;23:1639–1644.
68. Sowers MR, Wallace RB, Lemke JH. The association of intakes of vitamin D and calcium with blood pressure among women. *Am J Clin Nutr.* 1985;42:135–142.
69. Pfeifer M, Begerow B, Minne HW, Nachtigall D, Hansen C. Effects of a short-term vitamin D_3 and calcium supplementation on blood pressure and parathyroid hormone levels in elderly women. *J Clin Endocrinol Metab.* 2001;86:1633–1637.
70. Jorde R, Bonaa KH. Calcium from dairy products, vitamin D intake, and blood pressure: The Tromso study. *Am J Clin Nutr.* 2000;71:1530–1535.
71. Wang L, Manson JE, Buring JE, Lee IM, Sesso HD. Dietary intake of dairy products, calcium, and vitamin D and the risk of hypertension in middle-aged and older women. *Hypertension.* 2008;51:1073–1079.
72. Hsia J, Heiss G, Ren H, et al. Calcium/vitamin D supplementation and cardiovascular events. *Circulation.* 2007;115:846–854.
73. Li YC, Kong J, Wei M, Chen ZF, Liu SQ, Cao LP. 1.25-dihydroxyvitamin D_3 is a negative endocrine regulator of the renin-angiotensin system. *J Clin Invest.* 2002;110:229–238.
74. Shan J, Resnick LM, Lewanczuk RZ, Karpinski E, Li B, Pang PK. 1,25-dihydroxyvitamin D as a cardiovascular hormone. Effects on calcium current and cytosolic free calcium in vascular smooth muscle cells. *Am J Hypertens.* 1993;6:983–988.
75. Klar J, Sigl M, Obermayer B, Schweda F, Krämer BK, Kurtz A. Calcium inhibits renin gene expression by transcriptional and posttranscriptional mechanisms. *Hypertension.* 2005;46:1340–1346.
76. Richart T, Li Y, Staessen JA. Renal versus extrarenal activation of vitamin D in relation to atherosclerosis, arterial stiffening, and hypertension. *Am J Hypertens.* 2007;20:1007–1015.
77. Spies TD. Production of nonfatal vascular sclerosis in rabbits by means of viosterol (irradiated ergosterol). *Arch Int Med.* 1932;50:443–449.
78. Atkinson J, Poitevin P, Chillon JM, Lartaud I, Levy B. Vascular Ca overload produced by vitamin D3 plus nicotine diminishes arterial distensibilty in rats. *Am J Physiol.* 1994;266:H540–H547.
79. Holick MF. Vitamin D status: Measurement, interpretation and clinical application. *Ann Epidemiol.* 2009;19:73–78.
80. Lee JH, O'Keefe JH, Bell D, Hensrud DD, Holick MF. Vitamin D deficiency an important, common, and easily treatable cardiovascular risk factor? *J Am Coll Cardiol.* 2008;52:1949–1956.
81. Institute of Medicine. *Dietary Reference Intakes for Calcium and Vitamin D.* Washington, DC: The National Academies Press; 2011.
82. Carr AC, Frei B. Toward a new recommended dietary allowance for vitamin C based on antioxidant and health effects in humans. *Am J Clin Nutr.* 1999;69:1086–1107.
83. Jacques PF. The potential preventive effects of vitamins for cataract and age-related macular degeneration. *Int J Vitam Nutr Res.* 1999;69:198–205.
84. Hemila H. Vitamin C intake and susceptibility to the common cold. *Br J Nutr.* 1997;77:59–72.
85. Eriksson J, Kohvakka A. Magnesium and ascorbic acid supplementation in diabetes mellitus. *Ann Nutr Metab.* 1995;39:217–223.

86. Ness AR, Chee D, Elliott P. Vitamin C and blood pressure: An overview. *J Hum Hypertens.* 1997;11:343–350.
87. McRae MP. Is vitamin C an effective antihypertensive supplement? A review and analysis of the literature. *J Chiropr Med.* 2006;5:60–64.
88. Mullan BA, Young IS, Fee H, McCance DR. Ascorbic acid reduces blood pressure and arterial stiffness in type 2 diabetes. *Hypertension.* 2002;40:804–809.
89. Gokce N, Keaney JF Jr, Frei B, et al. Long-term ascorbic acid administration reverses endothelial vasomotor dysfunction in patients with coronary artery disease. *Circulation.* 1999;99:3234–3240.
90. Taddei S, Virdis A, Ghiadoni L, Magagna A, Salvetti A. Vitamin C improves endothelium-dependent vasodilation by restoring nitric oxide activity in essential hypertension. *Circulation.* 1998;97:2222–2229.
91. Sherman DL, Keaney JF Jr, Biegelsen ES, Duffy SJ, Coffman JD, Vita JA. Pharmacological concentrations of ascorbic acid are required for the beneficial effect on endothelial vasomotor function in hypertension. *Hypertension.* 2000;35:936–941.
92. Massey LK, Liebman M, Kynast-Gales SA. Ascorbate increases human oxaluria and kidney stone risk. *J Nutr.* 2005;135:1673–1677.
93. Levine M, Conry-Cantilena C, Wang Y, et al. Vitamin C pharmacokinetics in healthy volunteers: Evidence for a recommended dietary allowance. *Proc Natl Acad Sci USA.* 1996;93:3704–3709.
94. Rimm EB, Stampfer MJ, Ascherio A, Giovannucci E, Colditz GA, Willett WC. Vitamin E consumption and the risk of coronary heart disease in men. *N Engl J Med.* 1993;328:1450–1456.
95. Stampfer MJ, Hennekens CH, Manson JE, Colditz GA, Rosner B, Willett WC. Vitamin E consumption and the risk of coronary heart disease in women. *N Engl J Med.* 1993;328:1444–1449.
96. The Heart Outcomes Prevention Evaluation Study Investigators. Vitamin E supplementation and cardiovascular events in high-risk patients. *N Engl J Med.* 2000;342:154–160.
97. GISSI-Prevenzione investigators. Dietary supplementation with n-3 polyunsaturated fatty acids and vitamin E after myocardial infarction: Results of the GISSI-Prevenzione trial. *Lancet.* 1999;354:447–455.
98. Lonn EM, Yusuf S, Dzavik V, et al. Effects of ramipril and vitamin E on atherosclerosis: The study to evaluate carotid ultrasound changes in patients treated with ramipril and vitamin E (SECURE). *Circulation.* 2001;103:919–925.
99. Miller ER 3rd, Pastor-Barriuso R, Dalal D, Riemersma RA, Appel LJ, Guallar E. Meta-analysis: High-dosages vitamin E supplementation may increase all-cause mortality. *Ann Intern Med.* 2005;142:37–46.
100. Boshtam M, Rafiei M, Sadeghi K, Sarraf-Zadegan N. Vitamin E can reduce blood pressure in mild hypertensives. *Int J Vitam Nutr Res.* 2002;72:309–314.
101. Palumbo G, Avanzini F, Alli C. Effects of Vitamin E on clinic and ambulatory blood pressure in treated hypertensive patients. *Am J Hypertens.* 2000;13:564–567.
102. Pfeiffer CM, Caudill SP, Gunter EW, Osterloh J, Sampson EJ. Biochemical indicators of B vitamin status in the US population after folic acid fortification: Results from the National Health and Nutrition Examination Survey 1999–2000. *Am J Clin Nutr.* 2005;82:442–450.
103. Rader JI, Schneeman BO. Prevelence of neural tube defects, folate status, and folate fortification of enriched cereal-grain products in the United States. *Pediatrics.* 2006;117:1394–1399.

104. Homocysteine Studies Collaboration. Homocysteine and risk of ischemic heart disease and stroke: A meta-analysis. *JAMA.* 2002;228:2015–2022.
105. Ridker PM, Manson JE, Buring JE, Shih J, Matias M, Hennekens CH. Homocysteine and risk of cardiovascular disease among postmenopausal women. *JAMA.* 1999;281:1817–1821.
106. Tanne D, Haim M, Goldbourt U, et al. Prospective study of serum homocysteine and risk of ischemic stroke among patients with preexisting coronary heart disease. *Stroke.* 2003;34:632–636.
107. Welch GN, Loscalzo J. Homocysteine and atherothrombosis. *N Engl J Med.* 1998;338:1042–1050.
108. Brattstrom L, Wilcken DEL. Homocysteine and cardiovascular disease: Cause or effect? *Am J Clin Nutr.* 2000;72:315–323.
109. Brouwer IA, van Dusseldorp M, Thomas CM, et al. Low-dose folic acid supplementation decreases plasma homocysteine concentrations: A randomized trial. *Am J Clin Nutr.* 1999;69:99–104.
110. Jacques PF, Selhub J, Bostom AG, Wilson PW, Rosenberg IH. The effect of folic acid fortification on plasma folate and total homocysteine concentrations. *N Engl J Med.* 1999;340:1449–1454.
111. Lonn E, Yusuf S, Arnold MJ, et al. Homocysteine lowering with folic acid and B vitamins in vascular disease. *N Engl J Med.* 2006;354:1567–1577.
112. Bonaa KH, Njølstad I, Ueland PM, et al. Homocysteine lowering and cardiovascular events after myocardial infarction. *N Engl J Med.* 2006;354:1578–1588.
113. Albert CM, Cook NR, Gaziano JM, et al. Effect of folic acid and B-vitamins on risk of cardiovascular events and total mortality among women at high risk for cardiovascular disease: A randomized trial. *JAMA.* 2008;299:2027–2036.
114. Bazzano LA, Reynolds K, Holder KN, He J. Effect of folic acid supplementation on risk of cardiovascular diseases: A meta-analysis of randomized controlled trials. *JAMA.* 2006;296:2720–2736.
115. Wang X, Qin X, Demirtas H, et al. Efficacy of folic acid supplementation in stroke prevention: A meta-analysis. *Lancet.* 2007;369:1876–1882.
116. Ulrich CM. Folate and cancer prevention: A closer look at a complex picture. *Am J Clin Nutr.* 2007;86:271–273.
117. Van Dijk RA, Rauwerda JA, Steyn M, Twisk JW, Stehouwer CD. Long-term homocysteine-lowering treatment with folic acid plus pyridoxine is associated with decreased blood pressure but not with improved brachial artery endothelium-dependent vasodilation or carotid artery stiffness: A 2-year, randomized, placebo-controlled trial. *Arterioscler Thromb Vasc Biol.* 2001;21:2072–2079.
118. Mangoni AA, Sherwood RA, Swift CG, Jackson SH. Folic acid enhances endothelial function and reduces blood pressure in smokers: A randomized controlled trial. *J Intern Med.* 2002;252:497–503.
119. Cagnacci A, Cannoletta M, Volpe A. High-dose short-term folate administration modifies ambulatory blood pressure in postmenopausal women: A placebo-controlled study. *Eur J Clin Nutr.* 2009;63:1266–1268.
120. Forman JP, Rimm EB, Stampfer MJ, Curhan GC. Folate intake and the risk of incident hypertension among U.S. women. *JAMA.* 2005;293:320–329.
121. Forman JP, Stampfer MJ, Curhan GC. Diet and lifestyle risk factors associated with incident hypertension in women. *JAMA.* 2009;302:401–411.
122. de Bree A, van Faassen EE, Yo M, et al. Folic acid improves vascular reactivity in humans: A meta-analysis of randomized controlled trials. *Am J Clin Nutr.* 2007;86:610–617.

123. Stroes ES, van Faassen EE, Yo M, et al. Folic acid reverts dysfunction of endothelial nitric oxide synthase. *Circ Res.* 2000;86:1129–1134.
124. Doshi SN, McDowell IF, Moat SJ, et al. Folic acid improves endothelial function in coronary artery disease via mechanisms largely independent of homocysteine lowering. *Circulation.* 2002;105:22–26.
125. AACC report. The definition of dietary fiber. *Cereal Foods World.* 2001;46(3):112–126.
126. Alamo K. Dietary intake of vitamins, minerals, and fiber of persons ages 2 months and over in the United States: Third National Health and Nutrition Examinations Survey, phase 1, 1988–91. *Adv Data.* 1994;258:1–28.
127. Marlett JA, McBurney MI, Slavin JL, American Dietetic Association. Position of the American Dietetic Association: Health implications of dietary fiber. *J Am Diet Assoc.* 2002;102:993–1000.
128. Pereira MA, O'Reilly E, Augustsson K, et al. Dietary fiber and risk of coronary heart disease: A pooled analysis of cohort studies. *Arch Intern Med.* 2004;164:370–376.
129. Liu S, Manson JE, Stampfer MJ, et al. Whole grain consumption and risk of ischemic stroke in women: A prospective study. *JAMA.* 2000;284:1534–1540.
130. Liu S, Manson JE, Stampfer MJ, et al. A prospective study of whole-grain intake and risk of type 2 diabetes mellitus in U.S. women. *Am J Public Health.* 2000;90:1409–1415.
131. Fukagawa NK, Anderson JW, Hageman G, Young VR, Minaker KL. High-carbohydrate, high-fiber diets increase peripheral insulin sensitivity in healthy young and old adults. *Am J Clin Nutr.* 1990;52:524–528.
132. Olson BH, Anderson SM, Becker MP, et al. Psyllium-enriched cereals lower blood total cholesterol and LDL cholesterol, but not HDL cholesterol, in hypercholesterolemic adults: Results of a meta-analysis. *J Nutr.* 1997;127:1973–1980.
133. Streppel MT, Arends LR, van't Veer P, Grobbee DE, Geleijnse JM. Dietary fiber and blood pressure: A meta-analysis of randomized placebo-controlled trials. *Arch Intern Med.* 2005;165:150–156.
134. Whelton SP, Hyre AD, Pedersen B, Yi Y, Whelton PK, He J. Effects of dietary fiber intake on blood pressure: A meta-analysis of randomized, controlled clinical trials. *J Hypertens.* 2005;23:475–481.
135. Howard BV, Van Horn L, Hsia J, et al. Low-fat dietary pattern and risk of cardiovascular disease: The Women's Health Initiative Randomized Controlled Dietary Modification Trial. *JAMA.* 2006;295:655–666.
136. Keys A. Serum cholesterol response to dietary cholesterol. *Am J Clin Nutr.* 1984;40:351–359.
137. Hu FB, Stampfer MJ, Manson JE, et al. Dietary fat intake and the risk of coronary heart disease in women. *N Engl J Med.* 1997;337:1491–1599.
138. Mozaffarian D, Katan MB, Ascherio A, Stampfer MJ, Willett WC. Trans fatty acids and cardiovascular disease. *N Engl J Med.* 2006;354:1601–1613.
139. Harris WS, Mozaffarian D, Rimm E, et al. Omega-6 fatty acids and risk for cardiovascular disease: A science advisory from the American Heart Association Nutrition Subcommittee of the Council on Nutrition, Physical Activity, and Metabolism; Council on Cardiovascular Nursing; and Council on Epidemiology and Prevention. *Circulation.* 2009;119:902–907.
140. Mata P, Alvarez-Sala LA, Rubio MJ, Nuño J, De Oya M. Effects of long-term monounsaturated- versus polyunsaturated-enriched diets on lipoproteins in healthy men and women. *Am J Clin Nutr.* 1992;55:846–850.

141. Reaven P, Parthasarathy S, Grasse BJ, Miller E, Steinberg D, Witztum JL. Effects of oleate-rich and linoleate-rich diets on the susceptibility of low density lipoprotein to oxidative modification in mildly hypercholesterolemic subjects. *J Clin Invest.* 1993;91:668–676.

142. Bang HO, Dyerberg J, Sinclair HM. The composition of the Eskimo food in Northwestern Greenland. *Am J Clin Nutr.* 1980;33:2657–2661.

143. Dietary supplementation with n-3 polyunsaturated fatty acids and vitamin E after myocardial infarction: Results of the GISSI-Prevenzione trial. Gruppo Italiano per lo Studio della Sopravvivenza nell'infarto miocardico. *Lancet.* 1999;354:447–455.

144. Daviglus ML, Stamler J, Orencia AJ, et al. Fish consumption and the 30-year risk of fatal myocardial infarction. *N Engl J Med.* 1997;336:1046–1053.

145. Gerster H. Can adults adequately convert alpha-linolenic acid (18:3n-3) to eicosapentaenoic acid (20:5n-3) and docosahexaenoic acid (22:6n-3)? *Int J Vitam Nutr Res.* 1998;68:159–173.

146. Nestel PJ. Fish oil and cardiovascular disease: Lipids and arterial function. *Am J Clin Nutr.* 2000;71(suppl):228S–231S.

147. Leaf A, Kang JX, Xiao YF, Billman GE. Clinical prevention of sudden cardiac death by n-3 polyunsaturated fatty acids and mechanism of prevention of arrhythmias by n-3 fish oils. *Circulation.* 2003;107:2646–2652.

148. Omura M, Kobayashi S, Mizukami Y, et al. Eicosapentaenoic acid (EPA) induces Ca^{2+}-independent activation and translocation of endothelial nitric oxide synthase and endothelium-dependent vasorelaxation. *FEBS Lett.* 2001;487:361–366.

149. James MJ, Gibson RA, Cleland LG. Dietary polyunsaturated fatty acids and inflammatory mediator production. *Am J Clin Nutr.* 2000;71(suppl):343S–348S.

150. Geleijnse JM, Giltay EJ, Grobbee DE, Donders AR, Kok FJ. Blood pressure response to fish oil supplementation: Metaregression analysis of randomized trials. *J Hypertens.* 2002;20:1493–1499.

151. Appel LJ, Miller ER 3rd, Seidler AJ, Whelton PK. Does supplementation of diet with "fish oil" reduce blood pressure? A meta-analysis of controlled clinical trials. *Arch Intern Med.* 1993;153:1429–1438.

152. Morris MC, Sacks F, Rosner B. Does fish oil lower blood pressure? A meta-analysis of controlled trials. *Circulation.* 1993;88:523–533.

153. Mozaffarian D, Rimm EB. Fish intake, contaminants, and human health: Evaluating the risks and the benefits. *JAMA.* 2006;296:1885–1899.

154. Hashimoto M, Hossain S, Yamasaki H, Yazawa K, Masumura S. Effects of eicosapentaenoic acid and docosahexaenoic acid on plasma membrane fluidity of aortic endothelial cells. *Lipids.* 1999;34:1297–1304.

155. Lund EK, Harvey LJ, Ladha S, Clark DC, Johnson IT. Effects of dietary fish oil supplementation on the phospholipids composition and fluidity of cell membranes from human volunteers. *Ann Nutr Metab.* 1999;43:290–300.

156. Psaltopoulou T, Naska A, Orfanos P, Trichopoulos D, Mountokalakis T, Trichopoulou A. Olive oil, the Mediterranean diet, and arterial blood pressure: The Greek European Prospective Investigation into Cancer and Nutrition (EPIC) study. *Am J Clin Nutr.* 2004;80:1012–1018.

157. Williams PT, Fortmann SP, Terry RB, et al. Associations of dietary fat, regional adiposity, and blood pressure in men. *JAMA.* 1987;257:3251–3256.

158. Grimsgaard S, Bonaa KH, Jacobsen BK, Bjerve KS. Plasma saturated and linoleic acids are independently associated with blood pressure. *Hypertension.* 1999;34:478–483.

159. Gross LS, Li L, Ford ES, Liu S. Increased consumption of refined carbohydrates and the epidemic of type 2 diabetes in the United States: An ecologic assessment. *Am J Clin Nutr.* 2004;79:774–779.

160. Wolever TM, Jenkins DJ, Jenkins AL, Josse RG. The glycemic index: Methodology and clinical implications. *Am J Clin Nutr.* 1991;54:846–854.

161. Ludwig DS. The glycemic index: Physiological mechanisms relating to obesity, diabetes, and cardiovascular disease. *JAMA.* 2002;287:2414–2423.

162. Pereira MA, Swain J, Goldfine AB, Rifai N, Ludwig DS. Effects of a low-glycemic load diet on resting energy expenditure and heart disease risk factors during weight loss. *JAMA.* 2004;292:2482–2490.

163. Pawlak DB, Kushner JA, Ludwig DS. Effects of dietary glycaemic index on adiposity, glucose homoeostasis, and plasma lipids in animals. *Lancet.* 2004;364:778–785.

164. Salmeron J, Manson JE, Stampfer MJ. Dietary fiber, glycemic load and risk on non-insulin dependent diabetes mellitus in women. *JAMA.* 1997;277:472–477.

165. Sameron J, Manson JE, Stampfer MJ, Colditz GA, Wing AL, Willett WC. Dietary fiber, glycemic load, and risk of NIDDM in men. *Diabetes Care.* 1997;20:545–550.

166. Meyer KA, Kushi LH, Jacobs DR Jr, Slavin J, Sellers TA, Folsom AR. Carbohydrates, dietary fiber, and incident type 2 diabetes in older women. *Am J Clin Nutr.* 2000;71:921–930.

167. Liu S, Manson JE, Stampfer MJ, et al. Dietary glycemic load assessed by food-frequency questionnaire in relation to plasma high-density-lipoprotein cholesterol and fasting plasma triacylglycerols in postmenopausal women. *Am J Clin Nutr.* 2001;73:560–566.

168. Liu S, Manson JE, Buring JE, Stampfer MJ, Willett WC, Ridker PM. Relation between a diet with a high glycemic load and plasma concentrations of high-sensitivity C-reactive protein in middle-aged women. *Am J Clin Nutr.* 2002;75:492–498.

169. Lefebvre PJ, Scheen AJ. The postprandial state and risk of cardiovascular disease. *Diabet Med.* 1998;15:S63–68.

170. Liu S, Willett WC, Stampfer MJ, et al. A prospective study of dietary glycemic load, carbohydrate intake, and risk of coronary heart disease in U.S. women. *Am J Clin Nutr.* 2000;71:1455–1461.

171. Halton TL, Willett WC, Liu S, et al. Low-carbohydrate-diet score and the risk of coronary heart disease in women. *N Engl J Med.* 2006;355:1991–2002.

172. Higginbotham S, Zhang ZF, Lee IM, et al. Dietary glycemic load and risk of colorectal cancer in the women's health study. *J Natl Cancer Inst.* 2004;96:229–233.

173. Michaud DS, Liu S, Giovannucci E, Willett WC, Colditz GA, Fuchs CS. Dietary sugar, glycemic load, and pancreatic cancer risk in a prospective study. *J Natl Cancer Inst.* 2002;94:1293–1300.

174. Elliott SS, Keim NL, Stern JS, Teff K, Havel PJ. Fructose, weight gain, and the insulin resistance syndrome. *Am J Clin Nur.* 2002;76:911–922.

175. Appel LJ, Sacks FM, Carey VJ, et al. Effects of protein, monounsaturated fat, and carbohydrates intake on blood pressure and serum lipids: Results of the OmniHeart randomized trial. *JAMA.* 2005;294:2455–2464.

176. Stamler J, Caggiula A, Grandits GA, Kjelsberg M, Cutler JA. Relationship to blood pressure of combinations of dietary macronutrients: Findings of the Multiple Risk Factor Intervention Trial (MRFIT). *Circulation.* 1996;94:2417–2423.

177. Brown IJ, Elliott P, Robertson CE, et al. Dietary starch intake of individuals and their blood pressure: The international study of macronutrients and micronutrients and blood pressure. *J Hypertens.* 2009;27:231–236.

178. Stamler J, Liu K, Ruth KJ, Pryer J, Greenland P. Eight-year blood pressure change in middle-aged men: Relationship to multiple nutrients. *Hypertension.* 2002;39:1000–1006.

179. Title LM, Cummings PM, Giddens K, Nassar BA. Oral glucose loading acutely attenuates endothelium-dependent vasodilation in healthy adults without diabetes: An effect prevented by vitamins C and E. *J Am Coll Cardiol.* 2000;36:2185–2191.

180. Kopp W. Pathogenesis and etiology of essential hypertension: Role of dietary carbohydrate. *Med Hypotheses.* 2005;64:782–787.

181. Sacks FM, Rosner B, Kass EH. Blood pressure in vegetarians. *Am J Epidemiol.* 1974;100:390–398.

182. Armstrong B, van Merwyk AJ, Coates H. Blood pressure in Seventh-Day Adventist vegetarians. *Am J Epidemiol.* 1977;105:444–449.

183. Hu FB, Stampfer MJ, Manson JE, et al. Dietary protein and risk of ischemic heart disease in women. *Am J Clin Nutr.* 1999;79:221–227.

184. Appel LJ. The effects of protein intake on blood pressure and cardiovascular disease. *Curr Opin Lipidol.* 2003;14:55–59.

185. Iso H, Stampfer MJ, Manson JE, et al. Prospective study of fat and protein intake and risk of intraparenchymal hemorrhage in women. *Circulation.* 2001;103:856–863.

186. Klahr S, Levey AS, Beck GJ, et al. The effects of dietary protein restriction and blood pressure control on the progression of chronic renal disease: Modification of Diet in Renal Disease Study Group. *N Engl J Med.* 1994;330:877–884.

187. Stamler J, Elliott P, Kesteloot H, et al. Inverse relation of dietary protein markers with blood pressure: Findings for 10,020 men and women in the INTERSALT study. INTERSALT Cooperative Research Group. INTERnational Study of SALT and Blood Pressure. *Circulation.* 1996;94:1629–1634.

188. Elliott P, Stamler J, Dyer AR, et al. Association between protein intake and blood pressure: The INTERMAP study. *Arch Intern Med.* 2006;166:79–87.

189. Geleijnse JM, Hollman PC. Flavonoids and cardiovascular health: Which compounds, what mechanisms? *Am J Clin Nutr.* 2008;88:12–13.

190. Hooper L, Kroon PA, Rimm EB, et al. Flavonoids, flavonoid-rich foods, and cardiovascular risk: A meta-analysis of randomized controlled trials. *Am J Clin Nutr.* 2008;88:38–50.

191. Stamler J, Brown IJ, Daviglus ML, et al. Glutamic acid, the main dietary amino acid, and blood pressure: The INTERMAP study (International Collaborative Study of Macronutrients, Micronutrients and Blood Pressure). *Circulation.* 2009;120:221–228.

192. Moncada S, Higgs A. The L-arginine-nitric oxide pathway. *N Engl J Med.* 1994;329:2002–2012.

193. Sved AF, Fernstrom JD, Wurtman RJ. Tyrosine administration reduces blood pressure and enhances brain norepinephrine release in spontaneously hypertensive rats. *Proc Natl Acad Sci USA.* 1979;76:3511–3514.

194. Sved AF, Van Itallie CM, Fernstrom JD. Studies on the antihypertensive action of L-tryptophan. *J Pharmacol Exp Ther.* 1982;221:329–333.

chapter six

Diets

The prior chapter reviewed important nutrients that affect blood pressure and cardiovascular disease. Although each has a unique contribution, the various blends found in foods are also important. Consuming wholesome foods is the best way to obtain sufficient nutrition, although there may be a role for supplementation too. There are many commercially available diet plans, some fads and others based on sound scientific data, yet they all seem to claim either weight loss, protection from cardiovascular disease, promotion of overall health, or a combination thereof. It is recommended that individuals choose a sound diet that makes common sense and also provides safe, adequate nutrition. The Dietary Guidelines for Americans is published every 5 years and its latest version was released in 2010. It is available for free on the Internet at www.health.gov/dietary-guidelines/dga2010/DietaryGuidelines2010.pdf. Despite its title, the recommendations apply to Americans and non-Americans alike. Its purpose is to educate policy makers, nutrition educators, nutritionists, and health care providers about healthy dietary and lifestyle measures. It promotes eating nutrient-dense foods, such as vegetables, fruits, whole grains, low-fat dairy products, lean meats, and lean poultry, and recommends avoidance of added sugars, detrimental fats, and salts. It also advises on healthy weight maintenance and adequate exercise. Although it claims not to provide an actual diet plan, it does recommend specific consumption patterns within each food group, mostly based on the Dietary Reference Intake (DRI) reports of the Institute of Medicine. Adherence to such a diet is associated with lower mortality rates.[1] Two popular diet plans, the U.S. Department of Agriculture (USDA) Food Patterns and the Dietary Approaches to Stop Hypertension (DASH) Eating Plan, also are endorsed.

U.S. Department of Agriculture (USDA) food patterns

The USDA Food Patterns is an eating plan that closely follows the recommendations of the Dietary Guidelines for Americans. It promotes a diet of grains, vegetables, fruits, low-fat milk products, lean meats, and beans. There is allowance for a small amount of discretionary calories, which can be used for added sugars and fats. When properly implemented, adequate nutrition can be achieved. The plan is somewhat complex, as it separates vegetables into subgroups by color, such as orange or dark green, and recommends different amounts of each. The grains also are divided into categories—whole and refined. Fortunately, an interactive planner is available on the Internet at www.ChooseMyPlate.gov (formally www.mypyramid.gov), which is easy to use and even entertaining. It is tailored to the individual based on age, gender, height, and weight, accounting for differing caloric and nutritional needs. With a little effort, a sound meal plan can be created that includes most-favored foods and can be printed for easy access. Suggestions for weight management and exercise also are provided. Although a motivated person can design an adequate eating plan, it is still advisable to obtain assistance from a knowledgeable nutritionist.

Dietary Approaches to Stop Hypertension (DASH) eating plan

The Dietary Approaches to Stop Hypertension (DASH) clinical trial[2] is an important study worth describing in detail. It was based on observations that vegetarian diets and higher intakes of certain nutrients—such as potassium, magnesium, and calcium—are associated with lower blood pressure. The effects of a wholesome diet consisting of specific portions of vegetables, fruits, low-fat dairy products, lean meats/poultry/fish, nuts, and fats/oils on blood pressure were compared with a typical American diet. The DASH diet is designed to provide nutritional intake at the 75th percentile for potassium, magnesium, and calcium. The control diet, similar to a typical American diet, provided these nutrients at only the 25th percentile. The initial study did not focus on sodium intake, including levels similar to the characteristically high amounts found in a typical American diet. Four large U.S.-city-based medical centers participated in enrolling study subjects. About 60% of subjects were black and gender was about equally proportioned. All subjects had either prehypertension or stage I hypertension. Inclusion criteria for blood pressure was a systolic blood pressure <160 mm Hg and a diastolic blood pressure of 80 to 95 mm Hg. People with diabetes, elevated cholesterol levels, recent cardiovascular events, obesity, kidney insufficiency, excessive alcohol use, or those taking prescribed blood pressure medications were excluded. From 1994 to 1996, 459 adults were enrolled. All subjects were fed the control diet during a 3-week run-in period. Thereafter, they were randomly assigned to groups for an 8-week trial of one of three diets: the control diet, a diet rich in fruits and vegetables, or a diet rich in fruits and vegetables plus low-fat dairy products (i.e., the DASH diet). Subjects on the DASH diet had significant and superior lowering of their blood pressure compared with those on either of the other diets—a decrease of 5.5/3.0 mm Hg versus the control-diet group. A significantly better response of 11.4/5.5 mm Hg was observed for those with hypertension (i.e., a blood pressure of ≥140/90 mm Hg) and the response was even better for black subjects. These effects occurred within the first 2 weeks and persisted through the 8-week study period.

A second study published in 2001 compared the DASH diet at three levels of daily sodium intake: high (150 mmol or 3450 mg), intermediate (100 mmol or 2300 mg), and low (50 mmol or 1150 mg).[3] Sodium levels were based on a 2100 calorie per day diet and actual intake varied in proportion to the calorie needs of each subject. For example, a large male requiring a diet of 2600 calories per day would receive 124 mmol (2850 mg) rather than 100 mmol (2300 mg). An additional reduction of 3.0/1.6 mm Hg was observed between the high- and low-sodium intake groups. Larger effects were seen in subjects with hypertension, in black people, and in women. Overall, adherence to the DASH diet with sodium restriction had a better effect on hypertension than most blood pressure medications and could obviate the need for medication in many people. Adherence to the DASH diet also is associated with a lowered risk of future cardiovascular events and stroke.[4]

Details of the DASH Eating Plan are described in a publication called "Your Guide To Lowering Your Blood Pressure with DASH," which is available on the Internet at www.nhlbi.nih.gov/health/public/heart/hbp/dash/new_dash.pdf. The DASH diet is simpler than the USDA food guide and can be implemented by filling out the guidance tables provided in the publication. Sample menus are also available. Nonetheless, some direction from a knowledgeable nutritionist is recommended.

Mediterranean diet

The Mediterranean diet has been practiced in its native locale for thousands of years and more recently has been adopted worldwide. Although all countries along the Mediterranean Sea technically consume a Mediterranean diet, the term refers to the diets of Greece and southern Italy, circa 1960. An astute American physician, Ancel Keys, recognized an association between local diets of various countries and the prevalence of heart disease. He led a pioneering epidemiology study, The Seven Countries Study, which followed overall mortality rates, the mortality rates from heart disease, and the incidence of heart disease in men in seven countries starting in 1958. In 1970, detailed results were presented in a series of publications in the journal *Circulation*.[5] A clear relationship between diet—specifically saturated fat intake—and cholesterol levels, mortality rates, and the incidence of heart disease was observed. This connection was particularly evident in the Greek islands of Crete and Corfu where longevity and a lack of heart disease were apparent despite inferior medical care. It was speculated that their diet—the Mediterranean diet, rich in fruits, vegetables, unrefined cereals, dairy products, wine, and olive oil—contributed to these outcomes. Unfortunately, they also succumbed to the tribulations of modernity and presently consume a more Western-style diet. A subsequent study called the Lyon Diet Heart Study randomly assigned people with known heart disease to either a Mediterranean-type diet or to a "prudent" cardiovascular diet. The protective effects of the Mediterranean diet were so robust that the study was terminated early on ethical grounds, as it would have been unfair to continue the other diet.[6,7] Although many books have been published on its benefits, ideals, and practical implementation, the Mediterranean diet pyramid is perhaps the best known and highly regarded. It is sponsored by a joint effort from a nonprofit organization called Oldways, the Harvard School of Public Health, and the European Office of the World Health Organization. They present a variation of the Mediterranean diet from the 1960s and have updated this food guide at several dedicated conferences since 1995. The guideline is available on the Internet at www.oldwayspt.org/mediterranean-diet-pyramid. The initial plan and the subsequent modifications are based mostly on data from respected medical journals. In summary, it suggests a wholesome diet with abundant fruits, vegetables, tubers, whole grains, fish, dairy products, nuts, legumes, and seeds. Olive oil is central to the diet, conferring both rich flavor and beneficial fat. Wine is also an essential part of the plan. Eggs can be consumed but meats only in small portions, preferably poultry or lean red meat. Sweets also can be consumed in small amounts. There is an emphasis on enjoyment from food, both in its preparation and social interaction, which will further augment adherence to the diet. Adequate weight control and physical activity are also encouraged.

Recent studies have confirmed that adherence to a Mediterranean-type diet is associated with lower overall mortality rates from cardiovascular and cancer causes.[8,9] Improved blood lipid levels also have been noted.[10] The risk of developing diabetes,[11] several types of cancer,[12,13] and even Alzheimer disease[14] is also minimized. Blood pressure and hypertension rates are also lower in adherents of this food plan.[15] A systolic/diastolic blood pressure reduction of 3/2 mm Hg may occur in the general population,[16] with a larger effect in people with hypertension.[10] Consumption of olive oil is a major contributing factor to the blood pressure lowering effect.[17] Overall, this diet has many merits as well as being palatable and enjoyable.

Paleolithic diet

The Paleolithic diet, also called the hunter-gatherer diet, is a plan based on the presumed diet of human ancestry from the late Paleolithic period (about 10,000 years ago). The rationale is that during this era the human genome optimally adapted to this diet and that our genome today has not significantly changed. The diet consists of foods typically eaten by a hunter-gatherer society including meats, seafood, fruits, vegetables, nuts, and eggs. Foods such as dairy products, grains, legumes, salt, added sugars, and processed oils are excluded, because they mostly have been introduced in the subsequent Neolithic era and the more recent Industrial Revolution, when agrarian and livestock farming began and then became mechanized. Many variations of the Paleolithic diet exist with some even including dairy products; several texts are available, each describing its own version. Although there is sound scientific support for this diet, it is often considered a fad diet even by respected institutions such as the American Dietetic Association. Observational studies of modern hunter-gatherer societies such as the inhabitants of Kitava, New Guinea, suggest low rates of cardiovascular disease and stroke.[18] Insulin resistance also may be improved with this diet.[19] Results of a small study of 9 healthy people who consumed a Paleolithic diet for 10 days suggest benefit in lowering blood pressure and cholesterol levels.[20] An estimated nutritional breakdown of the ancestral-Paleolithic diet consists of roughly equal caloric intake of fats, proteins, and carbohydrates,[21] in contrast to the relatively high-carbohydrate diet of modern Western society. It also contains relatively high amounts of fiber, vitamins, and potassium, and low levels of sodium. These factors likely contribute to its presumed beneficial effects. Despite its Bohemian appeal it seems a difficult diet to adhere to and more clinical research is needed.

Atkins diet (very low-carbohydrate diet)

Low-carbohydrate diets have been practiced for well over a hundred years. Every few decades a new variation becomes popular, the most recent being the Atkins diet. Dr. Robert Atkins wrote several books for the general public. He explains its scientific basis as a very low-carbohydrate diet that causes the body to utilize fat stores instead of glucose, resulting in an increased basal metabolic rate, lower insulin blood levels, and production of ketones from fat metabolism. Some refer to this diet as a low-carbohydrate ketogenic diet.

Basically, the diet promotes fat metabolism while preserving muscle mass. It permits nondiscretional consumption of fats and proteins, while claiming significant weight loss and improved cardiovascular health. Blood lipid levels also are improved with increased HDL (high-density lipoprotein) and decreased triglyceride levels. Compared with a standard low-fat and calorie-restricted diet, several short-term studies confirm these claims,[22,23] although the effects may disappear within 12 months.[24] Improved control of diabetes[25] and of endothelial function[26] also have been demonstrated. Yet, despite the popularity and seeming success of the Atkins diet, it has been a source of much controversy, often vociferous. Dr.

Dean Ornish claims that comparison of the Atkins diet to conventional low-fat diets, which contain about 30% of calories from fat, is not a fair test.[27] Instead, he advocates a very low-fat diet comprised of <10% of vegetable-based fats along with other healthy lifestyle measures such as exercise and meditation. Direct comparison between the Ornish and Atkins diets is equivocal, with variable study results.[28,29] A significant problem with most of these studies is poor adherence, with up to 50% of participants dropping out. Furthermore, confirmation of dietary adherence is uncertain because study subjects are generally only questioned about it, as direct observation would be impossible in long-term studies. Therefore, these studies may not accurately reflect the true benefits and detriments of the diets. A serious concern with the Atkins diet had been reports of sudden cardiac death, likely due to electrolyte deficiencies as potassium and magnesium stores may become depleted. In one notable case report, a healthy teenager died shortly after starting the diet.[30] Another report described a healthy middle-aged man who developed impaired blood lipid levels, erectile dysfunction, and coronary atherosclerosis within a few years of starting the diet. Other studies suggest possible harmful effects from ketone production; these compounds may serve as precursors to substances such as methylglyoxal, which cause blood vessel and tissue damage.[31] Some feel the success of the diet is simply due to a decreased total calorie intake, since appetite is suppressed and many foods are restricted.[32] Other untoward side effects include halitosis, muscle cramps, and diarrhea. Despite all the criticism directed at Dr. Atkins, both in life and posthumously, one must admire his pioneering spirit and enthusiasm as well as the fact that many millions have benefited from his work.

The effects of a low-carbohydrate diet on blood pressure are less clear as few studies have addressed this topic. Of course, any weight loss would be associated with a lowering of blood pressure. A common comparison is between low-carbohydrate and low-fat diets with several studies showing a minimal lowering of systolic/diastolic blood pressure of up to 2 mm Hg with both types of diets.[22,28] However, other studies show a significantly better effect with the low-carbohydrate diet achieving reductions of 6–7/4–5 mm Hg.[29,33] It appears that there is a greater effect when weight loss is achieved through a low-carbohydrate diet. Possible mechanisms may involve lower blood insulin levels, which have a diuretic effect, and reduced sympathetic nervous system activity.[34]

South Beach diet (low-carbohydrate diet)

The South Beach diet was designed by Dr. Arthur Agatston, a cardiologist in the South Beach section of Miami Beach, Florida. Although originally designed as a diet to improve cardiovascular risk factors such as blood lipid levels, it quickly became a popular weight-loss diet. Although Dr.

Agatston firmly asserts that it is not a low-carbohydrate diet, despite few limitations on carbohydrate intake, it actually is one. It is not as extreme as the Atkins diet and the level of carbohydrate consumption is sufficient to avoid ketosis, although case reports of ketosis nonetheless exist,[35] especially during the initial phase. Although the initial phase is quite restrictive of carbohydrates and is similar to the Atkins diet, it only lasts for 2 weeks and thereafter becomes more liberal. The diet has no restrictions on total calorie intake but provides guidelines and examples of recommended dishes. Similar to the Atkins diet, it suggests low-glycemic-index foods, although unlike the Atkins diet it specifically recommends consumption of healthy fats such as monounsaturated and omega-3 fats and limited intake of saturated and trans fats. There are no limitations on the amounts of food consumed, based on the assumption that eating wholesome foods would lead to better satiety and consequent limits on total food intake. It is a sensible diet that promotes healthy eating habits through enjoyment of food and even anticipates the inevitable cheating, which is likely the beginning of the end of most diets. People seem to be able to successfully maintain this diet for lengthy periods, which is perhaps its most important quality.

Compared with the abundance of studies of very low-carbohydrate diets, relatively few exist for the South Beach diet. A short, 12-week study comparing the South Beach diet with a standard low-fat diet showed superior weight loss and favorable blood lipid levels with the former.[36] Debate over the cardiovascular benefits of a low-carbohydrate versus a low-fat diet seems perpetual. The most important factor in any diet is probably the amount of weight lost, which has a favorable effect on blood lipid levels. Nonetheless, a low-carbohydrate diet seems to more efficiently lower triglyceride levels, raise HDL cholesterol levels, and increase cholesterol particle size, all of which presumably improve cardiovascular health. However, in fairness, lower triglyceride levels may be due to lower overall insulin levels, and higher HDL cholesterol levels may simply be the body's response to increased fat intake and the need to process these products. Neither of these effects may confer improved cardiovascular health and may simply be byproducts of the diet itself. In fact, no comparative long-term study on the effects of a low-carbohydrate diet on cardiovascular health is yet available, and despite seemingly improved blood lipid levels, there is no conclusive proof that it results in truly important cardiovascular benefit. There also is experimental evidence that a low-carbohydrate diet may actually promote atherosclerosis and heart disease by mechanisms independent of blood lipids.[37] Furthermore, the Ornish diet, which is a very low-fat vegetarian diet containing <10% of daily calories from fat, is associated with significant reductions in LDL (low-density lipoprotein) cholesterol, improved coronary vessel patency, and cardiac viability.[38,39] Unfortunately, many find this diet too restrictive and adherence rates are poor.

In summary, the choice of diet type is rather complicated in the face of numerous commercially available options. The diet market is a multi-billion dollar a year business leading to the possible skewing of clarity in presentation of data and in recommendations. Perhaps the wisest choice is to adhere to the national guidelines but to aim for the lower end of carbohydrate intake of 45% of total calories. Of course, consumption of wholesome carbohydrates with low-glycemic indices, lean meats, and healthy fats is recommended.

References

1. Kant AK, Graubard BI, Schatzkin A. Dietary patterns predict mortality in a national cohort: The National Health Interview Surveys, 1987 and 1982. *J Nutr.* 2004;134:1793–1799.
2. Appel LJ, Moore TJ, Obarzanek E, et al. A clinical trial of the effects of dietary patterns on blood pressure. DASH Collaborative Research Group. *N Engl J Med.* 1997;336:1117–1124.
3. Sacks FM, Svetkey LP, Vollmer WM, et al. Effects on blood pressure of reduced dietary sodium and the Dietary Approaches to Stop Hypertension (DASH) diet. *N Engl J Med.* 2001;344:3–10.
4. Fung TT, Chiuve SE, McCullough ML, Rexrode KM, Logroscino G, Hu FB. Adherence to a DASH-style diet and risk of coronary heart disease and stroke in women. *Arch Intern Med.* 2008;168:713–720.
5. Coronary heart disease in seven countries. I. The study program and objectives. *Circulation.* 1970;41(4S1):I1–I8.
6. de Lorgeril M, Renaud S, Mamelle N, et al. Mediterranean alpha-linolenic acid-rich diet in secondary prevention of coronary heart disease. *Lancet.* 1994;343:1454–1459.
7. de Lorgeril M, Salen P, Martin JL, Monjaud I, Delaye J, Mamelle N. Mediterranean diet, traditional risk factors, and the rate of cardiovascular complications after myocardial infarction: Final report of the Lyon Diet Heart Study. *Circulation.* 1999;99:779–785.
8. Mitrou PN, Kipnis V, Thiébaut AC, et al. Mediterranean dietary pattern and prediction of all-cause mortality in a US population: Results from the NIH-AARP Diet and Health Study. *Arch Intern Med.* 2007;167:2461–2468.
9. Sofi F, Cesari F, Abbate R, Gensini GF, Casini A. Adherence to Mediterranean diet and health status: Meta-analysis. *BMJ.* 2008;337:a1344.
10. Estruch R, Martínez-González MA, et al. Effects of a Mediterranean-style diet on cardiovascular risk factors: A randomized trial. *Ann Intern Med.* 2006;145:1–11.
11. Martinez-Gonzalez MA, de la Fuente-Arrillaga C, Nunez-Cordoba JM, et al. Adherence to Mediterranean diet and risk of developing diabetes: Prospective cohort study. *BMJ.* 2008;336:1348–1351.
12. Benetou V, Trichopoulou A, Orfanos P, et al. Conformity to traditional Mediterranean diet and cancer incidence: The Greek EPIC cohort. *Br J Cancer.* 2008;99:191–195.
13. La Vecchia C, Bosetti C. Diet and cancer risk in Mediterranean countries: Open issues. *Public Health Nutr.* 2006;9:1077–1082.

14. Scarmeas N, Luchsinger JA, Schupf N, et al. Physical activity, diet, and risk of Alzheimer disease. *JAMA*. 2009;302:627–37.

15. Panagiotakos DB, Pitsavos CH, Chrysohoou C, et al. Status and management of hypertension in Greece: Role of the adoption of a Mediterranean diet: The Aticca study. *J Hypertens*. 2003;21:1483–1489.

16. Nunez-Cordoba JM, Valencia-Serrano F, Toledo E, Alonso A, Martínez-González MA. The Mediterranean diet and incidence of hypertension: The Seguimiento Universidad de Navarra (SUN) Study. *Am J Epidemiol*. 2009;169:339–346.

17. Psaltopoulou T, Naska A, Orfanos P, Trichopoulos D, Mountokalakis T, Trichopoulou A. Olive oil, the Mediterranean diet, and arterial blood pressure: The Greek European Prospective Investigation in Cancer and Nutrition (EPIC) Study. *Am J Clin Nutr*. 2004;80:1012–1018.

18. Lindeberg S, Lundh B. Apparent absence of stroke and ischaemic heart disease in a traditional Melanesian island: A clinical study in Kitava. *J Intern Med*. 1993;233:269–275.

19. Lindeberg S, Eliasson M, Lindahl B, Ahrén B. Low serum insulin in traditional Pacific Islanders: The Kitava Study. *Metabolism*. 1999;48:1216–1219.

20. Frassetto LA, Schloetter M, Mietus-Synder M, Morris RC Jr, Sebastian A. Metabolic and physiologic improvements from consuming a paleolithic, hunter-gatherer type diet. *Eur J Clin Nutr*. 2009;63:947–955.

21. Eaton SB. The ancestral human diet: What was it and should it be a paradigm for contemporary nutrition? *Proc Nutr Soc*. 2006;65:1–6.

22. Samaha FF, Iqbal N, Seshadri P, et al. A low-carbohydrate as compared with a low-fat diet in severe obesity. *N Engl J Med*. 2003;348:2074–2081.

23. Brehm BJ, Seeley RJ, Daniels SR, D'Alessio DA. A randomized trial comparing a very low carbohydrate diet and a calorie-restricted low fat diet on body weight and cardiovascular risk factors in healthy women. *J Clin Endocrinol Metab*. 2003;88:1617–1623.

24. Foster GD, Wyatt HR, Hill JO, et al. A randomized trial of a low-carbohydrate diet for obesity. *N Engl J Med*. 2003;348:2082–2090.

25. Nielsen JV, Joensson E. Low-carbohydrate diet in type 2 diabetes. Stable improvement of body weight and glycemic control during 44 months follow-up. *Nutr Metab (London)*. 2008;5:14.

26. Volek JS, Ballard KD, Silvestre R, et al. Effects of dietary carbohydrate restriction versus low-fat diet on flow-mediated dilation. *Metabolism*. 2009;58:1769–1777.

27. Ornish D. Was Dr. Atkins right? *J Am Diet Assoc*. 2004;104:537–542.

28. Dansinger ML, Gleason JA, Griffith JL, Selker HP, Schaefer EJ. Comparison of the Atkins, Ornish, Weight Watchers, and Zone diets for weight loss and heart disease risk reduction: A randomized trial. *JAMA*. 2005;293:43–53.

29. Gardner CD, Kiazand A, Alhassan S, et al. Comparison of the Atkins, Zone, Ornish, and LEARN diets for change in weight and related risk factors among overweight premenopausal women: The A to Z Weight Loss Study: A randomized trial. *JAMA*. 2007;297:969–977.

30. Stevens A, Robinson DP, Turpin J, Groshong T, Tobias JD. Sudden cardiac death of an adolescent during dieting. *South Med J*. 2002;95:1047–1049.

31. Beisswenger BG, Delucia EM, Lapoint N, Sanford RJ, Beisswenger PJ. Ketosis leads to increased methylglyoxal production on the Atkins diet. *Ann NY Acad Sci*. 2005;1043:201–210.

32. Astrup A, Meinert Larsen T, Harper A. Atkins and other low-carbohydrate diets: Hoax or an effective tool for weight loss? *Lancet.* 2004;364:897–899.

33. Yancy WS Jr, Westman EC, McDuffie JR, et al. A randomized trial of a low-carbohydrate diet versus orlistat plus a low-fat diet for weight loss. *Arch Intern Med.* 2010;170:136–145.

34. Passa P. Hyperinsulinemia, insulin resistance and essential hypertension. *Horm Res.* 1992;38:33–38.

35. Chalasani S, Fischer J. South Beach Diet associated ketoacidosis: A case report. *J Med Case Reports.* 2008;2:45.

36. Aude YW, Agatston AS, Lopez-Jimenez F, et al. The national cholesterol education program diet vs. a diet lower in carbohydrates and higher in protein and monounsaturated fat: A randomized trial. *Arch Intern Med.* 2004;164:2141-2146.

37. Smith SR. A look at the low carbohydrate diet. *N Engl J Med.* 2009;361:2286–2288.

38. Ornish D, Scherwitz LW, Billings JH, et al. Intensive lifestyle changes for reversal of coronary heart disease. *JAMA.* 1998;280:2001–2007.

39. Gould KL, Ornish D, Scherwitz L, et al. Changes in myocardial perfusion abnormalities by positron emission tomography after long-term, intense risk factor modification. *JAMA.* 1995;274:894–901.

chapter seven

Physical activity, relaxation techniques, and acupuncture

Physical activity

The health benefits of physical activity far outweigh possible harmful effects. Muscular and skeletal injuries are the most common complications, which fortunately can be avoided with proper safety and warm-up techniques. Less common, although more serious, are cardiac events, including sudden cardiac death and myocardial infarction, both more commonly associated with vigorous physical activity. However, the overall risk of sudden cardiac death is quite low, occurring in less than one per million episodes of vigorous exertion and even less frequently in those who are physically fit and who engage in regular vigorous physical activity.[1] Myocardial infarction, although a more common event, also occurs less frequently in physically fit people and in those who regularly engage in vigorous physical activity. Unfortunately, society has progressively become more sedentary, a problem of particular concern in adolescents.[2] This lifestyle may be responsible for as many as one-third of deaths due to coronary heart disease.[3]

The field of physical activity has become quite scientific and exacting. Although commonly viewed as any type of exercise, the definition of physical activity is far more complex. The U.S. Department of Health and Human Services (HHS) published the 2008 Physical Activity Guidelines for Americans,[4] which is available on the Internet at www.health.gov/paguidelines. Although intended for health care professionals, it is written for anyone to understand and can be applied to everyone. In promoting health benefits, HHS recommends specific prescriptions of physical activity based on age and physical conditioning. The recommendations are similar to those of the American College of Sports Medicine and the American Heart Association.[5] Physical activity is defined as any bodily movement due to muscular contraction that raises the energy expenditure of the body above that of its baseline and resting level (i.e., when quietly sitting). Exercise is a subcategory of physical activity performed to improve or maintain physical fitness, performance, or health. Examples of exercise include sports such as basketball or activities such as leisure walking. A construction worker's activity would not be considered exercise, although it is a form of physical activity.

Three types of physical activity are commonly referred to in the medical literature: aerobic, muscle strengthening, and bone strengthening. Examples of aerobic activity include walking, running, bicycling, and swimming. Muscle-strengthening activity, which primarily promotes muscle strength and mass, includes weight lifting, training with resistance bands, and calisthenics. Bone-strengthening activity, which promotes bone strength through impact forces, includes walking, running, and weight lifting. Physical activity can be classified within a single type or a combination thereof. For example, walking is a form of both aerobic and bone-strengthening activity. Although all three types of activity contribute to health maintenance, aerobic physical activity is the most important. The intensity of aerobic activity is graded in terms of metabolic equivalents (METs), which describe the energy expenditure of that particular activity. One MET equals the energy expenditure at rest (i.e., while sitting). Activities such as walking at a rate of 5 kilometers (3 miles) per hour requires 3 METs of energy, whereas running 10 kilometers (6 miles) per hour requires 6 METs. Aerobic activity is divided into subgroups: light intensity (1.0–2.9 METs), moderate intensity (3.0–5.9 METs), and vigorous intensity (6.0 and above METs). Tables for various aerobic physical activities and their corresponding METs are available.[5] Although this division of intensity is scientifically accurate, it is not practical, as people cannot easily convert their physical exertion into METs and then into its corresponding intensity subgroup. Therefore, the 2008 Physical Activity Guidelines for Americans adopted a relative intensity scale for physical activity based on a person's ability to perform. Using a scale of 0 to 10, where 0 is the level of effort at rest and 10 is the maximum effort, the subgroups are divided as follows: 1–4 = light-intensity physical activity; 5–6 = moderate intensity; and 7–10 = vigorous intensity. For most people, the relative scale roughly corresponds to the absolute scale using METs. However, for those who are very physically fit, the relative scale underestimates the absolute intensity of the activity. Similarly, it overestimates the absolute intensity for those with poor physical fitness, such as the elderly or chronically ill. Nonetheless, the guidelines apply the relative intensity scale to all people.

Most studies of the health effects of physical activity focus on the aerobic subtype. Habitual engagement in physical activity is associated with a lower risk of mortality[6,7] and with an adequate amount may prolong life by as much as 4 years in those over 50 years of age.[8] Vigorously intense activity may confer added longevity benefit.[9] The risk of cardiovascular disease is reduced[10,11] and there is also additional cardiovascular benefit to vigorous physical activity.[12] Blood lipid profiles are improved, with decreases in low-density lipoprotein (LDL) cholesterol and triglyceride levels and increases in high-density lipoprotein (HDL) cholesterol.[13,14] In addition, the particle sizes of the LDL and HDL cholesterol molecules are larger, which confers added benefit. Endothelial function is also improved.[15,16] Physical activity enhances the immune system, although acute bouts of vigorous exercise such as marathon running may temporarily reduce resistance.[17] Various malignancy rates such as for colon, liver, pancreas, stomach, and breast cancer are attenuated.[18–20] Insulin sensitivity is improved[21] and the risk of developing diabetes is reduced.[22] Cognitive decline and progression to dementia in the elderly is slowed[23,24] and the status of those with already impaired cognition can even be improved with physical activity.[25]

The role of physical activity in altering blood pressure has particular significance. Habitual aerobic physical activity may lower the resting (i.e., nonexercised) systolic/diastolic blood pressure by 5–7/4–6 mm Hg in people with hypertension and 3–4/2 mm Hg in those without hypertension.[26,27] Although the typical land-based types of aerobic activities such as walking, running, and bicycling are more popular, swimming has comparable benefits[28] and is especially appealing to those unable to adequately engage in higher-impact activities. Muscle-strengthening physical activity such as weightlifting also lowers resting blood pressure.[29] Although there is an immediate response within the first few days of training, most of the antihypertensive effect is not fully realized until about the 10th week.[30] Higher-intensity activity does not seem to have an added effect,[31] although this is debated.[32] Habitual physical activity can even prevent the onset of hypertension.[33,34]

The mechanisms by which physical activity lowers blood pressure are quite complex and not entirely clear, but several of its components are worth describing. Figure 7.1 is a schematic that describes some of the involved processes and humoral substances. Overall, blood pressure is lowered by both reduction in sympathetic nervous system activity and in blood plasma volume. Suppression of the sympathetic nervous system is evident by lower levels of norepinephrine. Several substances have been shown to suppress norepinephrine production and release. Prostaglandin E levels are elevated in people who regularly exercise and these hormones block release of norepinephrine mediated by the sympathetic nervous system.[35] Levels of the amino acid taurine also are elevated and have been shown to block norepinephrine release.[36] Through improved insulin sensitivity and reduced blood insulin levels, norepinephrine levels may also be suppressed.[37] Blood plasma volume, causing a reduced cardiac output and blood pressure, is also reduced with physical activity. The neurotransmitter dopamine is elevated in the early stages of exercise training and, through a diuretic effect, likely contributes to reducing blood plasma volume.[38] Another interesting humoral substance called ouabain may be involved. Ouabain has similar properties to the medicine digoxin and was traditionally used by African tribesmen in hunting wild game as injection

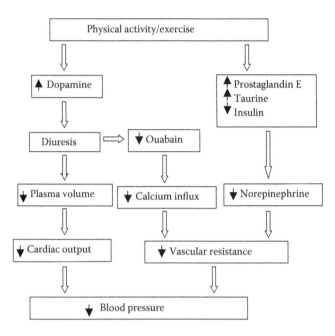

Figure 7.1 Mechanism of physical activity mediating reduction in blood pressure.

of the substance into prey (via an arrow tip) causes respiratory and cardiac paralysis. In therapeutic doses, it has several cardiac benefits and is also believed to be importantly involved in blood pressure regulation. It acts as a diuretic by blocking the sodium pumps in the kidney tubules, causing loss of sodium and water.[39] However, it also nonselectively blocks the sodium pumps of other cells, such as the vascular smooth muscle, resulting in increased or trapped intracellular sodium levels. Efforts to rid sodium from these cells utilize a sodium–calcium channel within the cell wall, causing exchange of sodium for calcium and consequent elevation of intracellular calcium. As previously described, elevated intracellular calcium levels cause constriction of the vascular smooth muscle cells and result in blood pressure elevation. In hypertension, especially salt-mediated hypertension, levels of ouabain are increased despite its vasoconstrictive and prohypertensive effects, probably in an effort to eliminate excess sodium and water. However, ouabain levels are suppressed with diuresis, achieved either through medicines or exercise-induced dopamine release,[40] leading to dilation of the arterioles and reduced blood pressure. Plasma renin levels are mostly unchanged with physical activity despite a reduced blood pressure. An interesting finding is an attenuated exercise-mediated antihypertensive response in people with hypertension who have higher levels of renin (i.e., renin-mediated hypertension).[35,41] This is probably due to physical activity's primary volume-mediated effect in lowering blood pressure. Physical activity is a V (volume)-type method of treating hypertension.

The 2008 Physical Activity Guidelines for Americans recommends appropriate prescription of physical activity based on age and physical and medical status.[4] These guidelines are similar to those of the American College of Sports Medicine and the American Heart Association.[5] They are intended for all people 6 years of age and older. The minimum recommended amount of physical activity is 500 MET minutes each week, which is enough to achieve significant benefit in most of the health-related areas discussed earlier. Aerobic-type activity is the primary focus, although muscle- and bone-strengthening activities also are recommended. The intensity of physical activity can be determined with either the absolute scale using METs or with the relative scale measured from 0 to 10. The recommended minimum dose for adults between the ages of 18 and 64 years is 150 minutes (2 hours, 30 minutes) of moderate-intensity aerobic physical activity each week. Because vigorous-intensity aerobic physical activity is equivalent to twice that of moderate intensity, 75 minutes (1 hour, 15 minutes) of this activity each week would be sufficient. A combination of moderate- and vigorous-intensity physical activity also is acceptable as long as it adds up to the minimum required amount. For example, 1 hour of moderate-intensity physical activity and 45 minutes of vigorous-intensity physical activity would suffice. Of course, additional activity is preferred as health benefits continue to accrue. It should be spread through at least 3 days of the week and each interval should last for at least 10 minutes. Routine office physical activity, such as walking up a few flights of stairs or intermittently carrying objects, does not count toward this total. Moderate- or high-intensity muscle-strengthening activities, which work most muscle groups of the body, should also be done at least twice a week. The guidelines for adults aged 65 and older are the same as for younger adults, although care should be taken in those with physical or medical limitations so as not to exceed their level of fitness. Balance-improving exercises should be done in individuals at risk of falling. Pregnant women also should perform at least 150 minutes of aerobic physical activity each week, but should avoid exercises requiring lying on the back. Children and adolescents require significantly higher doses of physical activity, which is probably the reason they were made with so much innate energy. A minimum of 60 minutes (1 hour) of either moderate- or vigorous-intensity aerobic physical activity each day is suggested, with the latter being included on at least 3 of these days. Playground activities such as running, hopping, and jumping rope are acceptable forms of aerobic exercise. Muscle-strengthening activities, such as climbing trees or playing tug-of-war, should be performed on at least 3 days of the week as part of the 60-minute total. Bone-strengthening activities such as playing basketball or running also should be included at least 3 times a week. Of course, these recommendations are the minimum prescribed dose and adding time will garner further health benefits.

Relaxation therapy

Psychosocial stress significantly affects our emotional and physical state of well-being. It can arise from acute events such as job loss, family disturbances, or bereavement, or from chronic causes such as depression, anxiety disorders, phobias, or anger disorders. Psychosocial stress has medical consequences due to its strong correlation with cardiovascular disease and hypertension. Stress has significance even in early life because adverse childhood experiences such as abuse and neglect predict future risk of cardiovascular disease.[42] INTERHEART, a global study involving thousands of adults, showed a significant association between psychosocial stress and myocardial infarction.[43] Another example of a reported increase in cardiac events is occurring within a 50-mile radius of the World Trade Center during the months following the September 11, 2001, terrorist attack.[44] Increased risk of stroke also is associated with psychosocial stress,[45] and anxiety disorders such as phobic anxiety correlate with increased risk of developing cardiovascular disease.[46,47] Chronic depression is not only more common in people with cardiovascular disease but is also an independent risk factor for its development.[48] Propensity to anger also independently predicts cardiovascular disease.[49] Although acute stress events such as job loss may transiently elevate the blood pressure, they are not likely to cause chronic hypertension in the same way chronic stress does.[50]

It is assumed that promoting relaxation therapy would improve cardiovascular health and blood pressure would be lower. There are a variety of techniques that help to reduce stress and promote relaxation. They work primarily by maintaining a mental or physical focus on either an endogenous or exogenous object. Many techniques carefully regulate breathing patterns, which has an unusually potent effect. Some methods such as transcendental meditation, Zen yoga, and Hatha yoga have origins in ancient religious philosophy. Newer approaches, such as autogenic training and progressive relaxation, focus on body awareness and relaxation. Biofeedback is a unique method that combines relaxation techniques with various physical body inputs. An example is the use of a thermal finger sensor to feed information back to a person to induce relaxation. Fingertip temperature is a good marker of the degree of relaxation, as relaxation causes blood vessels to dilate with subsequent increase in blood flow to the fingertips and temperature elevation. As blood pressure also is reduced with vessel dilation, fingertip temperature is a good gauge of blood pressure as well. An individual can be trained to use these methods in conjunction with relaxation techniques in order to lower blood pressure. It usually requires significant work with a skilled biofeedback therapist and can take many sessions to master, although once learned can be done at home without the need for biofeedback input.

Despite the clear association of stress with cardiovascular disease and hypertension, evidence that relaxation therapy ameliorates these conditions is less convincing, although it probably is effective. Much of the ambiguity arises from lack of scientifically rigorous and long-term studies. A particular issue with blood pressure studies is the use of clinic or office blood pressure as the target measurement, as these studies are particularly prone to bias from a white-coat effect. Because this effect is a stress-mediated process, it is difficult to sort the true effects of relaxation therapy, as it may just be correcting a white-coat effect. Many studies provide clever sham therapies in the control group, but it is difficult to completely eliminate the effect. The use of ambulatory or home blood pressure monitoring would avoid this problem, but unfortunately few studies choose this as their end point. Despite the difficulties, the evidence is still convincing that relaxation therapy is protective of cardiovascular disease.[51–53] There is also evidence that it lowers blood pressure with a reduction of 5/3 mm Hg being shown in people with hypertension, although the true value would likely be smaller if adequate placebo and sham effects were taken into account.[54]

There is a unique device called the Resperate, which lowers blood pressure through breathing guided biofeedback. It does not require training with a professional as do other relaxation and biofeedback techniques and, unlike most other techniques, it has been studied with adequate controls. It is approved by the U.S. Food and Drug Administration (FDA) for treatment of hypertension. Respiration patterns and rates seem to be closely associated with psychosocial relaxation and consequently blood pressure. For this reason, many meditative techniques focus on breathing patterns. Respiration affects regional blood flow and blood pressure throughout the body, which varies during the different parts of the breathing cycle.[55] As mentioned in Chapter 2, blood pressure is regulated partly by input from various baroreceptors, which sense blood pressure changes, and from chemoreceptors, which sense changes in the levels of blood chemicals such as oxygen and carbon dioxide. These receptors are stimulated differently during the parts of the breathing cycle and they regulate the sympathetic nervous system, subsequently altering blood vessel tone and blood pressure. Slower respiration rates with a prolonged expiration phase cause reduction in sympathetic nervous system output and lower blood pressure. The Resperate device trains individuals to reduce their respiratory rates to less than 10 breaths per minute. A rate of 6 breaths per minute is of special significance as it may synchronize with the spontaneous fluctuation pattern of the baroreceptors and chemoreceptors, called Mayer waves. The components of the device include a belt with a respiration sensor that fits around the chest, a computer that senses the respiration rate, and a headphone that sends peaceful tones to the user to guide breathing rates and patterns. The computer generates varied pitched tones for inspiration and expiration and slowly trains users to prolong their expiration phase and slow their breathing rate. Suggested treatment comprises 15-minute sessions on most days of the week. Most of the effect on blood pressure occurs by the fourth week of use. The manufacturer claims a reduction in systolic/diastolic office blood pressure of 14/8 mm Hg in people with hypertension compared with 9/4 mm Hg in control groups. Home blood pressure is reduced by 5/3 mm Hg compared with no response in control groups.[56] The device can be purchased through the Internet and although somewhat expensive, it is cheaper than the multiple sessions of relaxation therapy needed to master other techniques and certainly cheaper than lifelong use of medication.

The mechanism by which relaxation therapy lowers blood pressure involves reduction in sympathetic nervous system output.[57] This causes dilation of the blood vessels and lowers levels of renin and aldosterone through decreased nervous system input to the kidneys and adrenal glands.[58] Therefore, it is a mixed V- and R (renin)-type method of lowering blood pressure. A major drawback of relaxation therapies is that many of the techniques are time consuming, requiring multiple and lengthy practice each day. Given the questionable benefit in lowering blood pressure along with the typical time constraints in modern society, it is difficult to recommend most of these techniques, especially if an individual uses them to replace efforts to achieve other goals such as healthy eating and adequate physical activity. The Resperate device is an exception as its benefit is more clearly proven and it only requires one short session several times a week, although more use would provide additional benefit.

Acupuncture

Acupuncture is a part of traditional Chinese medicine with origins as far back as 4000 years. It was codified in the medical text Haungdi Neijing, translated as "The Yellow Emperor's Inner Canon," written approximately in the 2nd century BCE. Although the form of acupuncture used today originated in China, there may have been coincidental use in both Europe and Egypt, as evidenced by specific skin markings found in well-preserved remains of people living in these regions as far back as 5000 years ago. The term "acupuncture" is derived from the Latin word *acu*, defined as "with a needle," and the English word *puncture*. Fine needles, usually made of stainless steel, are inserted under the skin at various locations in the body. Earlier forms of acupuncture used sharpened stone, bone, or bamboo. Variants of acupuncture include acupressure, electroacupuncture, moxibustion, and cupping. In moxibustion, dried moxa leaves are attached to the end of an acupuncture needle and then burned sending heat to the needle tip and adding efficacy. The theory behind acupuncture is quite detailed and of comparable complexity to Western medicine, requiring many years of study to understand and adequately master. According to traditional Chinese medicine, a ubiquitous life force known as chi, which is present throughout the world, is channeled through the body along linear tracks beneath the skin surface known as meridians. For example, the lung meridian starts at the shoulder and tracks down to the distal part of the thumb. The purpose of acupuncture is to restore the proper flow of chi in the meridians and the body, which is achieved by stimulating various acupuncture points along the meridians. There are 12 symmetric pairs of meridians and 2 additional unpaired ones. Each meridian is usually associated with a major organ, such as the lungs, the heart, and the kidneys. Chi is transferred to and from the organs via the meridians, somewhat analogous to the circulatory system that circulates blood. The meridians also have interconnecting points that allow chi to pass between them. There are different types of chi such as protective chi, harmful chi, nourishing chi, clean chi, and waste chi. Traditional Chinese medicine also assigns a yin or yang quality to chi, the meridians, and the body organs. A yin quality is often more docile, relating to elements such as cold and quiet, whereas a yang quality is hot and active. The health of a person is maintained by having proper balance of chi throughout the meridians and the body. When an imbalance occurs, such as from a disruption or deficiency of chi in a meridian, it can in itself cause illness or make the body more susceptible to harmful external chi and illness. Diagnosis of disease is important in traditional Chinese medicine and requires careful inspection of physical signs such as the character of the pulse and tongue, complexion, skin texture, voice, and odor. A detailed history of habits such as eating, sleeping, and body excretions is also sought. This is akin to the physical exam taught in Western medical schools, an underpracticed art. It is a truly holistic approach.

From the perspective of a Western-trained physician, the principles of traditional Chinese medicine may seem unreal. I admit these were my sentiments when first reading about acupuncture. However, it reminded me of an experience I had as a graduate student while studying toward my doctoral thesis. My research was in the field of laser spectroscopy and I studied the energy states of small radical molecules. As part of my dissertation, I built a machine called a photoelectron spectrometer, which measured the flow of electrons released from these molecules after being bombarded with a high-energy laser pulse. The test molecule was nitric oxide, as it had properties favorable for the calibration of the machine. I remember being struck by a sense of awe on the first day of successfully measuring these electron flows. After all, electrons are subatomic particles, which have never actually been seen or trapped. They are only part of a theoretical model, yet there they were appearing as a signal on my oscilloscope. In a similar way, the supernatural forces of traditional Chinese medicine are also part of a constructed theory and as acupuncture has helped billions of people spanning many generations and cultures, it too deserves credit and respect.

Although traditional Chinese medicine and acupuncture were first introduced into Western society in the 17th century, they did not become popular until the later part of the 20th century, in part due to the change in policy toward China initiated during the Nixon administration. The World Health Organization sponsored a multicultural seminar on acupuncture in 1979, which endorsed potential treatments of many illnesses including neurological, respiratory, gastrointestinal, and oral disorders, although these claims were based primarily on anecdotal experience rather than controlled clinical trials. In 1997, the National Institutes of Health sponsored a conference on the medical uses of acupuncture, which more carefully examined the medical literature.[59] They recognized an overall lack of adequate studies in support of efficacy for most illnesses treated by acupuncture, although there was sufficient evidence for treatment of nausea and dental pain. These findings led to recognition of the need for more scientific research into the efficacy of acupuncture. Although there are many Western medical studies supporting the role of acupuncture in treating pain disorders, there is a paucity of studies in support of treating cardiovascular disease. A few studies suggest improved symptoms in people with angina pectoris[60,61] and animal studies show improvement of myocardial ischemia.[62] The treatment of hypertension is better studied, as several large and credible studies are reported. Unfortunately, the findings are not consistent; some support the use of acupuncture to treat hypertension with a modest reduction in systolic/diastolic blood pressure of 6/4 mm Hg,[63] whereas others do not.[64,65] The effect also is not long lasting and the blood pressure tends to revert back to its original level without continued acupuncture treatments. Clearly, more clinical trials are still needed to determine a genuine effect.[66]

The mechanisms by which acupuncture regulates the cardiovascular system and treats pain probably involves enhanced production of brain opioids.[67] Two such opioid classes, the endorphins and the enkephalins, act on specific regions of the brain and reduce overall sympathetic nervous system output.[68] Studies show both increased nitric oxide levels[69] and reduced renin levels,[70] most likely due to direct reduction in sympathetic nervous system output. Consequent vasodilation of the vessels and reduced blood pressure then may occur. Acupuncture would therefore be a mixed V- and R-type method of lowering blood pressure. However, as the substantiating data of its efficacy in lowering blood pressure has not been clearly established in accord with Western scientific standards and its implementation is both costly and time consuming, it is difficult at this time to recommend its use in treating hypertension. Perhaps the main problem is in trying to characterize acupuncture in terms of Western medicine, which is like comparing apples with oranges. Still, it is a safe technique and billions of people seemed to have benefited from it.

References

1. Albert CM, Mittleman MA, Chae CU, Lee IM, Hennekens CH, Manson JE. Triggering of sudden death from cardiac causes by vigorous exertion. *N Engl J Med.* 2000;343:1355–1361.
2. Matthews CE, Chen KY, Freedson PS, et al. Amount of time spent in sedentary behaviors in the United States, 2003–2004. *Am J Epidemiol.* 2008;167:875–881.
3. Powell KE, Blair SN. The public health burdens of sedentary living habits: Theoretical but realistic estimates. *Med Sci Sports Exerc.* 1994;26:851–856.
4. US Department of Health and Human Services. 2008 Physical Activity Guidelines for Americans. http://www.health.gov/paguidelines. Accessed April 30, 2012.
5. Haskell WL, Lee IM, Pate RR, et al. Physical activity and public health: Updated recommendations for adults from the American College of Sports Medicine and the American Heart Association. *Circulation.* 2007;116:1081–1093.
6. Leitzmann MF, Park Y, Blair A, et al. Physical activity recommendations and decreased risk of mortality. *Arch Intern Med.* 2007;167:2453–2460.
7. Andersen LB, Schnohr P, Schroll M, Hein HO. All-cause mortality associated with physical activity during leisure time, work, sports, and cycling to work. *Arch Intern Med.* 2000;160:1621–1628.
8. Franco OH, de Laet C, Peeters A, Jonker J, Mackenbach J, Nusselder W. Effects of physical activity on life expectancy with cardiovascular disease. *Arch Intern Med.* 2005;165:2355–2360.
9. Lee IM, Hsieh CC, Paffenbarger RS Jr. Exercise intensity and longevity in men: The Harvard Alumni Health Study. *JAMA.* 1995;273:1179–1184.
10. Tanasescu M, Leitzmann MF, Rimm EB, Willett WC, Stampfer MJ, Hu FB. Exercise type and intensity in relation to coronary heart disease in men. *JAMA.* 2002;288:1994–2000.
11. Lee IM, Rexrode KM, Cook NR, Manson JE, Buring JE. Physical activity and coronary heart disease in women: Is "no pain, no gain" passé? *JAMA.* 2001;285:1447–1454.
12. Swain DP, Franklin BA. Comparison of cardioprotective benefits of vigorous versus moderate intensity aerobic exercise. *Am J Cardiol.* 2006;97:141–147.
13. Kraus WE, Houmard JA, Duscha BD, et al. Effects of the amount and intensity of exercise on plasma lipoproteins. *N Engl J Med.* 2002;347:1483–1492.
14. Halverstadt A, Phares DA, Wilund KR, Goldberg AP, Hagberg JM. Endurance exercise training raises high-density lipoprotein cholesterol and lowers small low-density lipoprotein and very low-density lipoprotein independent of body fat phenotypes in older men and women. *Metabolism.* 2007;56:444–450.
15. Hambrecht R, Wolf A, Gielen S, et al. Effect of exercise on coronary endothelial function in patients with coronary artery disease. *N Engl J Med.* 2000;342:454–460.
16. DeSouza CA, Shapiro LF, Clevenger CM, et al. Regular aerobic exercise prevents and restores age-related declines in endothelium-dependent vasodilation in healthy men. *Circulation.* 2000;102:1351–1357.

17. Shephard RJ, Shek PN. Exercise, immunity, and susceptibility to infection: A J-shaped relationship? *Phys Sportsmed*. 1999;27:47–71.
18. Inoue M, Yamamoto S, Kurahashi N, Iwasaki M, Sasazuki S, Tsugane S. Daily total physical activity level and total cancer risk in men and women: Results from a large-scale population-based cohort study in Japan. *Am J Epidemiol*. 2008;168:391–403.
19. Michaud DS, Giovannucci E, Willett WC, Colditz GA, Stampfer MJ, Fuchs CS. Physical activity, obesity, height, and the risk of pancreatic cancer. *JAMA*. 2001;286:921–929.
20. Rockhill B, Willett WC, Hunter DJ, Manson JE, Hankinson SE, Colditz GA. A prospective study of recreational physical activity and breast cancer risk. *Arch Intern Med*. 1999;159:2290–2296.
21. Mayer-Davis EJ, D'Agostino R Jr, Karter AJ, et al. Intensity and amount of physical activity in relation to insulin sensitivity: The Insulin Resistance Atherosclerotic Study. *JAMA*. 1998;279:669–674.
22. Hu FB, Sigal RJ, Rich-Edwards JW, et al. Walking compared with vigorous physical activity and risk of type 2 diabetes in women: A prospective study. *JAMA*. 1999;282:1433–1439.
23. Yaffe K, Barnes D, Nevitt M, Lui LY, Covinsky K. A prospective study of physical activity and cognitive decline in elderly women: Women who walk. *Arch Intern Med*. 2001;161:1703–1708.
24. Abbott RD, White LR, Ross GW, Masaki KH, Curb JD, Petrovitch H. Walking and dementia in physically capable elderly men. *JAMA*. 2004;292:1447–1453.
25. Lautenschlager NT, Cox KL, Flicker L, et al. Effect of physical activity on cognitive function in older adults at risk for Alzheimer disease: A randomized trial. *JAMA*. 2008;300:1027–1037.
26. Whelton SP, Chin A, Xin X, He J. Effect of aerobic exercise on blood pressure: A meta-analysis of randomized, controlled trials. *Ann Intern Med*. 2002;136:493–503.
27. Fagard RH. Physical activity in the prevention and treatment of hypertension in the obese. *Med Sci Sports Exerc*. 1999;31:S624–S630.
28. Tanaka H, Bassett DR Jr, Howley ET, Thompson DL, Ashraf M, Rawson FL. Swimming training lowers the resting blood pressure in individuals with hypertension. *J Hypertens*. 1997;15:651–657.
29. Kelley GA, Kelley KS. Progressive resistance exercise and resting blood pressure. A meta-analysis of randomized controlled trials. *Hypertension*. 2000;35:838–843.
30. Petrella RJ. How effective is exercise training for the treatment of hypertension? *Clin J Sport Med*. 1998;8:224–231.
31. Fagard RH. Exercise characteristics and the blood pressure response to dynamic physical training. *Med Sci Sports Exerc*. 2001;33:S484–S492.
32. Nemoto K, Gen-no H, Masuki S, Okazaki K, Nose H. Effects of high-intensity interval walking training on physical fitness and blood pressure in middle-aged and older people. *Mayo Clin Proc*. 2007;82:803–811.
33. Haapanen N, Miilunpalo S, Vuori I, Oja P, Pasanen M. Association of leisure time physical activity with risk of coronary heart disease, hypertension and diabetes in middle-aged men and women. *Int J Epidemiol*. 1997;26:739–747.
34. Hayashi T, Tsumura K, Suematsu C, Okada K, Fujii S, Endo G. Walking to work and the risk for hypertension in men: The Osaka Health Survey. *Ann Intern Med*. 1999;131:21–26.

35. Kiyonaga A, Arakawa K, Tanaka H, Shindo M. Blood pressure and hormonal responses to aerobic exercise. *Hypertension.* 1985;7:125–131.

36. Tanabe Y, Urata H, Kiyonaga A, et al. Changes in serum concentrations of taurine and other amino acids in clinical antihypertensive exercise therapy. *Clin Exp Hypertens A.* 1989;11:149–165.

37. Arakawa K. Effect of exercise on hypertension and associated complications. *Hypertens Res.* 1996;19:S87–S91.

38. Kinoshita A, Koga M, Matsusaki M, et al. Changes of dopamine and atrial natriuretic factor by mild exercise for hypertensives. *Clin Exp Hypertens A.* 1991;13:1275–1290.

39. Blaustein MP, Hamlyn JM. Sodium transport inhibition, cell calcium, and hypertension: The natriuretic hormone/NA+/Ca2+ exchange/hypertension hypothesis. *Am J Med.* 1984;77:45–59.

40. Koga M, Ideishi M, Matsusaki Site, et al. Mild exercise decreases plasma endogenous digitalis-like substance in hypertensive individuals. *Hypertension.* 1992;19(2 suppl):II231–II236.

41. Urata H, Tanabe Y, Kiyonaga A, et al. Antihypertensive and volume-depleting effects of mild exercise on essential hypertension. *Hypertension.* 1987;9:245–252.

42. Dong M, Giles WH, Felitti VJ, et al. Insights into causal pathways for ischemic heart disease: Adverse childhood experiences study. *Circulation.* 2004;110:1761–1766.

43. Rosengren A, Hawken S, Ounpuu S, et al. Association of psychosocial risk factors with risk of acute myocardial infarction in 11119 cases and 13648 controls from 52 countries (the INTERHEART study): Case-control study. *Lancet.* 2004;364:953–962.

44. Allegra JR, Mostashari F, Rothman J, Milano P, Cochrane DG. Cardiac events in New Jersey after September 11, 2001, terrorist attack. *J Urban Health.* 2005;82:358–363.

45. Ohlin B, Nilsson PM, Nilsson JA, Berglund G. Chronic psychosocial stress predicts long-term cardiovascular morbidity and mortality in middle-aged men. *Eur Heart J.* 2004;25:867–873.

46. Kawachi I, Colditz GA, Ascherio A. Prospective study of phobic anxiety and risk of coronary heart disease in men. *Circulation.* 1994;89:1992–1997.

47. Shen BJ, Avivi YE, Todaro JF, et al. Anxiety characteristics independently and prospectively predict myocardial infarction in men: The unique contribution of anxiety among psychologic factors. *J Am Coll Cardiol.* 2008;51:113–119.

48. Lichtman JH, Bigger JT Jr, Blumenthal JA, et al. Depression and coronary heart disease: Recommendations for screening, referral, and treatment: A science advisory from the American Heart Association Prevention Committee of the Council on Cardiovascular Nursing, Council on Clinical Cardiology, Council on Epidemiology and Prevention, and Interdisciplinary Council on Quality of Care and Outcomes Research: Endorsed by the American Psychiatric Association. *Circulation.* 2008;118:1768–1775.

49. Williams JE, Paton CC, Siegler IC, Eigenbrodt ML, Nieto FJ, Tyroler HA. Anger proneness predicts coronary heart disease risk: Prospective analysis from atherosclerosis risk in communities (ARIC) study. *Circulation.* 2000;101:2034–2039.

50. Sparrenberger F, Cichelero FT, Ascoli AM, et al. Does psychosocial stress cause hypertension? A systematic review of observational studies. *J Hum Hypertens.* 2009;23:12–19.

51. Patel C, Marmot MG, Terry DJ, Carruthers M, Hunt B, Patel M. Trial of relaxation in reducing coronary risk: Four-year follow-up. *Br Med J (Clin Res Ed)*. 1985;290:1103–1106.
52. Linden W, Stossel C, Maurice J. Psychosocial interventions for patients with coronary artery disease: A meta-analysis. *Arch Intern Med*. 1996;156:745–752.
53. van Dixhoorn J, White A. Relaxation therapy for rehabilitation and prevention in ischemic heart disease: A systematic review and meta-analysis. *Eur J Cardiovasc Prev Rehabil*. 2005;12:193–202.
54. Dickinson H, Campbell F, Beyer F, et al. Relaxation therapies for the management of primary hypertension in adults: A Cochrane review. *J Hum Hypertens*. 2008;22:809–820.
55. Parati G, Izzo JL, Gavish B. Respiration and blood pressure. In: Izzo JL, Sica DA, Black HR, eds. *Hypertension Primer: The Essentials of High Blood Pressure*. 4th ed. Philadelphia: Lippincott, Williams, and Wilkins; 2008:136–138.
56. Grossman E, Grossman A, Schein MH, Zimlichman R, Gavish B. Breathing-control lowers blood pressure. *J Hum Hypertens*. 2001;15:263–269.
57. Schwartz AR, Gerin W, Davidson KW, et al. Toward a causal model of cardiovascular responses to stress and the development of cardiovascular disease. *Psychosom Med*. 2003;65:22–35.
58. Patel C, Marmot MG, Terry DJ. Controlled trial of biofeedback-aided behavioral methods in reducing mild hypertension. *Br Med J (Clin Res Ed)*. 1981;282:2005–2008.
59. NIH Consensus Conference. Acupuncture. *JAMA*. 1997;15:1–34.
60. Richter A, Herlitz J, Hjalmarson A. Effect of acupuncture in patients with angina pectoris. *Eur Heart J*. 1991;12:175–178.
61. Ballegaard S, Jensen G, Pedersen F, Nissen VH. Acupuncture in severe, stable angina pectoris: A randomized trial. *Acta Med Scand*. 1986;220:307–313.
62. Li P, Pitsillides KF, Rendig SV, Pan HL, Longhurst JC. Reversal of reflex-induced myocardial ischemia by median nerve stimulation: A feline model of electroacupuncture. *Circulation*. 1998;97:1186–1194.
63. Flachskampf FA, Gallasch J, Gefeller O, et al. Randomized trial of acupuncture to lower blood pressure. *Circulation*. 2007;115:3121–3129.
64. Macklin EA, Wayne PM, Kalish LA, et al. Stop Hypertension with Acupuncture Research Program (SHARP): Results of a randomized, controlled clinical trial. *Hypertension*. 2006;48:838–845.
65. Robinson RC, Wang Z, Victor RG, et al. Lack of effect of repetitive acupuncture on clinic and ambulatory blood pressure. *Am J Hypertens*. 2004;17:33A.
66. Lee H, Kim SY, Park J, Kim YJ, Lee H, Park HJ. Acupuncture for lowering blood pressure: Systematic review and meta-analysis. *Am J Hypertens*. 2009;22:122–128.
67. Chao DM, Shen LL, Tjen-A-Looi S, Pitsillides KF, Li P, Longhurst JC. Naloxone reverses inhibitory effect of electroacupuncture on sympathetic cardiovascular reflex responses. *Am J Physiol*. 1999;276:H2127–H2134.
68. Napadow V, Ahn A, Longhurst J, et al. The status and future of acupuncture mechanism research. *J Altern Complement Med*. 2008;14:861–869.
69. Kim DD, Pica AM, Durán RG, Durán WN. Acupuncture reduces experimental renovascular hypertension through mechanisms involving nitric oxide synthases. *Microcirculation*. 2006;13:577–585.
70. Lee HS, Kim JY. Effects of acupuncture on blood pressure and plasma renin activity in two-kidney one clip Goldblatt hypertensive rats. *Am J Chin Med*. 1994;22:215–219.

chapter eight

Dietary (nonpharmaceutical) supplements

The role of dietary supplements in health maintenance has become prominent and regarded. They significantly add to the available methods of treating disease and in maintaining health. Its expanding scope is appreciated by the ever-increasing promotion in media outlets such as television, radio, and the Internet, and by anyone visiting their local pharmacy or vitamin superstore. The available products far outnumber the standard drugs used by clinicians. They are commonly promoted as natural and healthy alternatives to standard drugs. However, for several reasons, they should be regarded with caution. As opposed to standard drugs, they do not have the classification of pharmaceutical agents, and therefore in most countries are not regulated by governmental medical agencies. In the United States, they are not regulated by the Food and Drug Administration, which has rather strict guidelines for standard pharmaceutical products. As such, the quality of these products varies depending on the manufacturer, and often the labeled dose of the active ingredient is inaccurate. More concerning is contamination with toxic substances such as heavy metals. Lead, mercury, and arsenic are commonly found in Ayurvedic medicines[1] and various other toxins are well described.[2] Unfortunately, dietary supplements do not need to list these toxic components on their labels. Data from NHANES shows elevated levels of lead in those using herbal supplements.[3] Dietary supplements are often marketed as natural and therefore safe and healthy products, yet the doses of many extracts are equivalent to several folds, sometimes several thousand folds, the concentration of the product in its raw form. This clearly is not natural. Finally, for many products, the supporting scientific data is limited and often anecdotal. Fortunately, agencies such as the U.S. Pharmacopeial (USP) Verification Program verify the doses and safety of these products and it is advisable to use products under their supervision. They are clearly marked as "USP verified." Last, dietary supplements should be regarded, as suggested by its name, as supplements only. They are not a replacement to pharmaceutical agents or to healthy lifestyle and dietary measures.

This chapter will describe several well regarded dietary supplements, which have a reasonable breadth of supporting scientific evidence and time-honored use.

L-arginine

L-arginine is an amino acid found in human protein. It is considered a nonessential amino acid, as the body can synthesize adequate amounts, but a substantial amount is obtained from the diet as well. Although it is a constituent of protein, it is also a component of the urea cycle and serves as a precursor molecule in creatine synthesis. L-arginine is important to endothelial function as the sole precursor of nitric oxide (NO). Since the 1980s, NO has received much attention for its importance in human physiology. The Nobel Prize in medicine was awarded in 1998 to the researchers who first described its function.

Figure 8.1 describes the conversion of L-arginine to NO, which is catalyzed by the enzyme nitric oxide synthase (NOS). This process occurs in all cells, although is of particular importance in endothelial cells and the juxtaglomelular apparatus cells of the kidney. In human physiology, there are two types of endothelial NO synthases, eNOS and iNOS. The former is a constitutive enzyme that continuously produces low levels of NO independent of physiologic need, whereas iNOS is a high-flux enzyme that generates large amounts of NO and is present during states of stress and inflammation such as in atherosclerotic plaque or infection. NO also mediates vasodilation of the blood vessels and therefore has the potential to lower blood pressure.

Many have hypothesized that L-arginine supplementation will improve endothelial function, cardiovascular health, and lower blood pressure, largely through its ability to produce NO. Much research has been conducted, although the findings have been inconclusive and inconsistent. A possible explanation for these inconsistencies may be due to the types of people included in the studies, as some included healthy subjects and others included subjects with various cardiovascular risk factors and illness. A more consistent response to L-arginine supplementation is observed if studies are classified according to the level of endothelial dysfunction of its subjects. Division into three broad groups is sufficient: (1) healthy people with normal endothelial function; (2) people with mild-to-moderate endothelial dysfunction, such as those with hypertension, hypercholesterolemia, diabetes, mild coronary artery disease, and the elderly; and (3) people with severe endothelial dysfunction such as those with significant atherosclerosis or severe heart disease. Studies of healthy

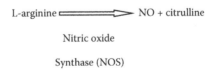

Figure 8.1 Nitric-oxide-synthase-mediated synthesis of nitric oxide.

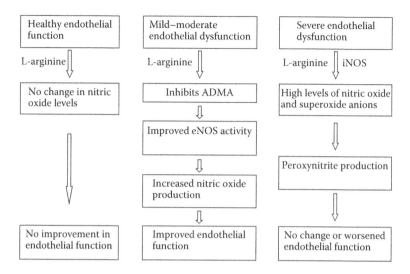

Figure 8.2 Effect of L-arginine on endothelial function.

individuals (group 1)[4,5] and of those with severe endothelial dysfunction (group 3)[6,7] often do not show benefit from L-arginine supplementation. However, individuals with mild-to-moderate endothelial dysfunction (group 2) have shown improved function and amelioration of their under-lying disease states in response to supplementation. Examples of group 2 populations that benefited are individuals with hypercholesterolemia,[8] relatively young people with stable coronary artery disease,[9] people with congestive heart failure but no signs of atherosclerosis or other cardiovas-cular risk factors,[10] and the elderly.[11] A description of the kinetic models of NO synthesis and the chemistry involved in endothelial dysfunction is needed to help appreciate these observations. Figure 8.2 describes the mechanisms involved. Surprisingly, there is an apparent excess of L-arginine within tissue, as its physiologic cellular concentration is about 25 to 30 times higher than the capacity of the enzyme eNOS to convert it to NO. Therefore, the limiting factor in NO production is from levels of the enzyme rather than the substrate. This may explain why healthy people with normal endothelial function do not benefit from L-arginine supplementation: they are already maximally producing NO. However, it does not explain why supplementation improves NO production and endothelial function in those with underlying endothelial dysfunction. This dilemma is known as the L-arginine paradox, because these indi-viduals also should be maximally producing NO. A possible explanation may come from involvement of a similar molecule called asymmetric dimethylarginine (ADMA). Because elevated levels of ADMA are found in disease states such as hypercholesterolemia, hypertension, kidney dis-ease, and cardiovascular disease, it is considered a marker of endothelial dysfunction.[12,13] It is a competitive inhibitor of the enzyme eNOS and therefore interferes with the conversion of L-arginine to NO. In disease states, where ADMA levels are elevated, the conversion rate of L-arginine to NO is slowed, causing further endothelial dysfunction. L-arginine is an antagonist of ADMA, suppressing its inhibitory effect on eNOS and consequently increasing NO production.[14] Therefore, in states of endothelial dysfunction that are worsened by ADMA, L-arginine may reverse the process. Although this may explain why L-arginine supplementation improves endothelial function in those with mild-to-moderate endothelial dysfunction, it does not explain the lack of improvement in those with more severe dysfunction. In fact, it even may be harmful, as reported in a study of people with recent myocardial infarction who had higher mortality rates after receiving L-arginine supplements.[7] A possible explanation may be that levels of iNOS, the other NO synthase, are increased in the endothelium of people with severe atherosclerosis and severe systemic inflammation.[15] Similar to eNOS, it converts L-arginine to NO and citrulline, but it achieves this conversion more rapidly and efficiently. This creates a milieu of high levels of NO and other toxic radicals, such as superoxide anion, in atherosclerotic plaque. This mix of radical molecules will form toxic peroxynitrites that promote local tissue damage and atherosclerosis and may even inactivate eNOS. Therefore, supplementation of L-arginine may cause too much NO production and cause untoward effects in states of severe endothelial dysfunction. An additional factor may be the synthesis of creatine, which also uses L-arginine as its precursor molecule and produces homocysteine as a byproduct; homocysteine itself may be an independent cardiovascular risk factor. In summary, this may explain why supplementation of L-arginine in states of severe endothelial dysfunction may not be beneficial and may even be harmful.

Based on this model, most people with hypertension who have mild-to-moderate endothelial dysfunction would benefit from L-arginine supplementation. There are only a few studies that measure the effects of such supplementation on blood pressure. Although some show blood pressure reduction in healthy people with normal blood pressure,[16] the effect is more pronounced in those with hypertension.[17,18] The primary mechanism of lowering blood pressure is vasodilation due to increased NO levels.[19] Additional contributions may arise from the effects of NO on the kidneys, specifically on the juxtaglomerular apparatus that regulates the tubuloglomerular feedback system and controls filtration rates[20] and the amount of tubular retention of salt and water,[21] which cause diuresis. A third, but less significant cause is inhibition of the angiotensin-converting enzyme (ACE).[22] NO also may have a minimal direct role in stimulating renin secretion.[23] Overall, L-arginine supplementation has minimal effect on renin levels[24,25] and is therefore a V (volume)-type method of treating hypertension.

Although L-arginine supplementation appears promising in treating hypertension, especially salt-mediated hypertension, a major drawback to its use is the need for daily intake of many pills to be effective. Studied doses vary from 9 to 21 grams a day, usually divided into three doses, and considering that each tablet is typically 500 mg this would require a patient to take 18 to 42 pills a day. Such high doses are needed because L-arginine has a short half-life (about 1 hour), and most of the drug is metabolized within a few hours. A sustained-released formulation is available, typically in a 350 mg tablet form, and the use of three tablets (1050 mg) twice daily has been shown to reduce systolic/diastolic blood pressure by 11/5 mm Hg in people with hypertension.[17] This would require taking six pills each day, which is still difficult to recommend as primary treatment. Increased dietary intake of L-arginine also has shown benefit.[16] Fish such as tuna and salmon have high levels as do nuts such as peanuts, almonds, sunflower seeds, and walnuts. Incorporation of these foods into the diet is good practice.

Coenzyme Q_{10}

Coenzyme Q_{10} (CoQ_{10}) is an endogenously produced substance. It is also called ubiquinone because of its ubiquitous presence in all human cells, mostly within the mitochondrial organelles. Its primary function is to facilitate electron transfer within the mitochondrial electron transport chain, making it an integral part of aerobic respiration and production of adenosine triphosphate (ATP). It is also an antioxidant and is protective of lipid peroxidation and from radical-induced degradation of cellular membranes, which cause atherosclerosis and endothelial dysfunction. It is produced in sufficient quantity in healthy people, and therefore is technically not a vitamin but rather a vitamin-like substance. Its synthesis shares precursor molecules and chemical pathways with cholesterol synthesis as these two substances are biologically linked. Therefore, CoQ_{10} deficiency may occur with use of statin drugs, which block both cholesterol and CoQ_{10} production,[26,27] although this finding is debated.[28] Levels also decrease with age[29] and with exposure to ultraviolet light and sunlight.[30]

The role of CoQ_{10} in health is mostly studied vis-à-vis its effects on cardiovascular disease. This is not surprising given its prominent role in aerobic respiration and its antioxidant properties. CoQ_{10} levels in heart tissue are reduced in people with heart disease, especially in those with advanced stages of heart failure.[31] Studies have shown benefit from its use as adjunctive therapy to conventional heart failure treatment. Improved clinical signs and symptoms such as reduced peripheral edema, pulmonary edema, insomnia, and palpitations,[32,33] as well as improved objective findings such as increases in cardiac output and cardiac ejection fraction[34] have been reported. However, other and perhaps more recent studies do not support these beneficial effects.[35,36] CoQ$_{10}$ supplementation is likely to benefit people with heart failure, although more convincing trials are still needed. Several small studies suggest a protective effect from angina symptoms.[37] Daily supplements following a myocardial infarction also may minimize the risk of subsequent cardiac events.[38] Tissue levels of CoQ$_{10}$ also may be reduced in people with hypertension.[39] Studies on the effect of CoQ$_{10}$ supplementation in hypertension appear to be more conclusive than the cardiovascular studies. Doses of about 100 mg per day may lower systolic/diastolic blood pressure by 11–17/7–10 mm Hg in people with hypertension.[40,41] CoQ$_{10}$ may also improve glycemic control in people with diabetes,[42] slow progression of symptoms in Parkinson's disease,[43] ameliorate the frequency and severity of migraine headaches,[44] and facilitate treatment of some cancers.[45]

The mechanisms in which CoQ$_{10}$ affects disease are multifactorial. As previously discussed, its primary function of enhancing aerobic respiration and ATP production helps in treating cardiac diseases. It also has antiradical properties that minimize lipid peroxidation and radical-induced degradation of cellular membranes that cause both atherosclerosis and endothelial dysfunction. Improved endothelial function contributes to its blood-pressure-lowering effect by causing vasodilation.[41] Plasma renin levels are not affected.[46] CoQ$_{10}$ supplementation is therefore a V-type method of treating hypertension.

The side effects of CoQ$_{10}$ supplementation are minimal, with mild gastrointestinal discomfort occurring in less than 1% of individuals.[47] Because reduced anticoagulant efficacy has been reported, it may be problematic in people taking warfarin (Coumadin),[48] and insufficient data is available to recommend its use in pregnant women or in children. A dose of 100 mg per day has been shown to be adequate in providing most cardiovascular and blood-pressure-lowering benefits, although higher doses may be needed to treat other diseases. It has a relatively long half-life, enabling once-daily dosing. CoQ$_{10}$ is poorly absorbed through the gastrointestinal tract because it has unfavorable water- and lipid-solubility properties. Several clever drug vehicle formulations are available, but perhaps the most efficient one is a type called Q-gel.[49] Although CoQ$_{10}$ can be obtained naturally from foods, specifically from meat, fish, and some oils, it would require excessive consumption to adequately replete tissue stores, as a typical dietary intake is only 3 to 6 mg per day.[50] Although blood serum levels can be measured in commercial laboratories, these values are of limited use because the true effect of CoQ$_{10}$ more accurately depends on tissue levels. For those with hypertension or heart disease, a reasonable daily supplementation is 100 mg. It takes from 4 to 12 weeks for its full effect to be realized. Despite being more effective in nonrenin-mediated hypertension, it can be recommended for everyone, given its relatively benign character and the fact that most hypertension is of a mixed renin and nonrenin type.

Garlic (Allium sativum)

Garlic has had rich societal, culinary, religious, and medicinal roles in many cultures over the centuries. Its use is noted in Sanskrit records from some 5000 years ago, and it plays an important role in traditional Chinese medicine as well as those of the ancient Egyptian, Greek, and Roman cultures. In the 19th century, Louis Pasteur observed an antibacterial effect of garlic and it was used as an antiseptic during World Wars I and II.[51] Since the 1960s, garlic has gained popularity in scientific research and a multitude of studies have been performed. Although it is highly touted for its cardiovascular benefits, relatively few studies directly examine its role in prevention and treatment of heart disease. Instead, most focus on cardiovascular risk factors such as cholesterol levels, fibrinolytic activity, platelet aggregation activity, atherosclerosis, diabetes, and hypertension. The majority of studies focus on lipid levels, and although results are mixed and often contradictory, garlic probably does lower total cholesterol, low-density lipoprotein (LDL) cholesterol, and triglyceride levels.[52,53] Increased fibrinolytic activity and decreased platelet aggregation also have been demonstrated,[52,53] which theoretically reduce atherosclerosis and acute cardiovascular events. Prevention and even regression of atherosclerosis has been shown as well.[54,55] Reduced risks of developing colorectal and stomach cancer[56,57] and even prevention of the common cold[58] have been suggested. Studies on the effect of garlic supplementation on blood pressure have mixed results, but there is a probable lowering effect in people with hypertension.[59,60] A reduction in systolic/diastolic pressure of 8–16/7–9 mm Hg has been reported,[59,60] which is comparable to most commercial medications, although the robustness of this claim is questionable. Much of the problem stems from a lack of studies of adequate scientific rigor and quality.[61] Equally important is a lack of uniformity in the type of garlic supplement used, as there are many formulations. It can be consumed raw or as commercial supplements such as garlic powder tablets, aged garlic extract (AGE), or various oil-based extract formulations. Garlic contains several putative biologically active agents, which differ in quantity depending on the supplement. Different types of garlic, such as wild versus cultivated garlic, also contain different ratios of these compounds. The most well-regarded active compound is a sulfur-based thiosulfinate called allicin, which is rapidly produced from the conversion of alliin by the enzyme alliinase (see Figure 8.3). Although many feel it is the most important active agent in garlic, this is questionable due to its very low bioavailability and the extensive degradation it undergoes in the liver prior to absorption into the circulation.[62] Other compounds such

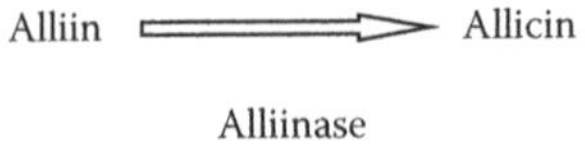

$$Alliin \rightleftharpoons Allicin$$

Alliinase

Figure 8.3 Alliinase-mediated synthesis of allicin.

as S-allylcysteine found in AGE also may contribute effect and may be more efficacious in lowering blood pressure and cholesterol levels.[52] For all these reasons, it is difficult to accurately determine the effect of garlic supplementation.

The mechanism by which garlic supplementation lowers blood pressure is multifaceted. It has been shown to inhibit ACE,[63] as well as to cause vasodilation via NO-dependent[64,65] and independent mechanisms.[66] It therefore has mixed R (renin)- and V-type properties in lowering blood pressure. Typical daily doses would be either 4 g (roughly two cloves) of raw garlic, which must be crushed or chewed; dried garlic tablets (typically 300 mg/1.3% alliin) taken three times daily; or 7.2 grams of AGE.[51] However, in light of all the misgivings it is difficult to recommend it as a primary treatment of hypertension.

Polyphenols

Polyphenols are a group of organic-chemical compounds found in plants. Several hundred have been identified in edible plants, although many more exist within the plant kingdom.[67] They have many biological and medicinal effects, in part due to their antioxidant properties and involvement in enzymatic processes. Historically, they have not received the regard given to vitamins and minerals, although they are slowly gaining acceptance as an important part of the diet. Four groups of polyphenols, based on chemical structure, are of importance: the flavonoids, the stilbenes, the phenolic acids, and the lignans. Within each group there are many subgroups of individual molecules. Lists of polyphenol contents for individual foods are available, although their accuracy is uncertain because the amounts may vary depending on factors such as location of harvest, type of cultivation, and degree of ripeness. Furthermore, differences in digestive ability and types of food preparations (e.g., cooking and processing) also alter its bioavailability. It is difficult, therefore, to characterize the contribution of polyphenol to health. Among the polyphenol groups, the flavonoids have received the most attention and often serve as a representative of all polyphenols with regard to medical benefit. Several well-regarded studies have suggested their consumption provides protection from cardiovascular disease[68–70] and stroke.[71] Despite further classification into individual molecules, most medical studies focus on specific foods, which are often rich in various types of polyphenols. Soy protein, cocoa, tea, and red wine are a few of the more often-cited foods, each representing a unique blend of polyphenol compounds, and a review of them is worthwhile.

Soy protein

Soy protein is a good source of a flavonoid subgroup called the isoflavones. It contains three important isoflavone compounds—genistein, daidzein, and glycitein—although a fourth compound called equol is produced from daidzein by the microflora (bacteria) in the intestines (Figure 8.4). Soy protein and the isoflavones have received much attention relating to their ability to modify cardiovascular risk factors. Observational studies in Japan and other Asian countries, where large amounts of soy are consumed, show reduced rates of cardiovascular disease. The isoflavones are structurally similar to estrogen and can bind to estrogen receptors at physiologic doses. A prevalent theory is that pro-estrogen effects are in part responsible for these results, similar to the beneficial effects of hormone replacement therapy. Modification of cholesterol levels is the most commonly studied parameter and an important meta-analysis from 1995 suggested ingestion of soy protein results in large reductions in LDL, triglycerides, and total cholesterol levels.[72] Based on these preliminary observations the FDA, in 1999, approved the labeling of foods with soy protein as being protective of coronary heart disease. In 2000, the American Heart Association (AHA) also recommended its consumption. However, several studies since then have reported more modest reduction in cholesterol levels,[73,74] and some even suggest that the isoflavones are not even the active ingredients in soy protein.[75] Other theories suggest that the unique mix of amino acids or the specific amino acid sequences within soy protein are the causative factors.[76] This led the AHA to modify its statement about the benefits of soy protein in 2006.[77] Aside from effects on cholesterol levels, soy protein and isoflavones also have been associated with prevention of LDL oxidation,[78] reduced platelet aggregation,[79] and diminished rates of atherosclerosis in animal studies.[80] Protection from breast cancer[81] and amelioration of hot flushes in postmenopausal women[82] also have been reported.

Studies of soy intake on blood pressure show varied results ranging from robust effects[83,84] to none at all.[85] There is likely a small lowering

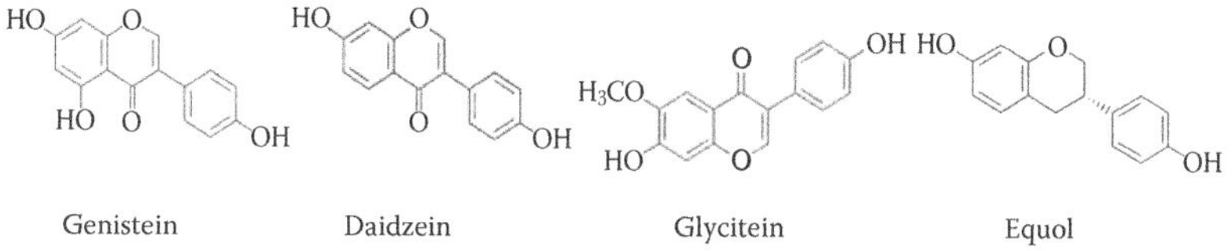

Genistein   Daidzein   Glycitein   Equol

Figure 8.4 Active polyphenol molecules in soy protein.

of systolic/diastolic blood pressure of about 3/2 mm Hg, from either soy protein isolate or isoflavone extract.[86] A larger reduction may be expected in people with hypertension. Mechanisms by which soy reduces blood pressure include inhibition of ACE,[87] diuresis,[88] and vasodilation via production of NO.[89] No clearly dominant pathway is yet characterized and therefore soy protein consumption is considered a mixed R- and V-type method of lowering blood pressure. A significant drawback observed in most studies is that large quantities of soy protein, typically 50 g a day, were consumed in order to confer benefit. For many people this equates to more than half of their daily protein intake, and especially in Western society where soy consumption is less common, this is not a reasonable expectation. As such, and given its modest medical effects, it is difficult to recommend soy protein as a primary treatment for hypertension.

Chocolate (cocoa, cacao)

Chocolate has important cultural and medicinal functions spanning many centuries and countries. Its origins are in the Mesoamerica region (roughly defined as Central America) with evidence of use some 3000 years ago by the Olmec civilization and subsequently by the Mayans and the Aztecs.[90] With the Spanish conquest of the New World in the 16th century, it was introduced to Spain, and thereafter gained popularity throughout Europe. Although often used interchangeably, cacao, cocoa, and chocolate are actually distinct foods. Cacao is the partially processed seed of the theobroma cacao tree, consisting of both cocoa butter and cocoa solids. Cocoa is usually referred to as the solid or powder component of cacao, and chocolate itself is a mix of various proportions of cocoa butter and cocoa solids. The ancient Mesoamerican cultures consumed the beverage cacao, which in its natural form is quite bitter, unlike the often-sweetened forms adopted by Western society. The processing of cacao to modern-day chocolate involves many steps that alter its nutrient content, making today's product quite different from the traditional cacao beverage.

Chocolate is a good source of a flavonoid subgroup called the flavanols. Two flavanols, epicatechin and catechin, and their oligomers (i.e., larger molecules composed of several of these units linked together) are particularly abundant, and these compounds are considered to be the active medicinal components of chocolate (Figure 8.5). As the processing of chocolate alters the flavanol content, it is instructive to understand these steps. Each cacao pod has many beans (or seeds) with surrounding pulp. The beans are separated and allowed to ferment—an important step in enhancing flavor. The beans are then dried, the pulp removed, and the beans roasted and cracked open to allow the inner part, called nibs, to be removed. Nibs are often sold in health food stores and contain roughly equal portions of cocoa solids and cocoa butter. The nibs are ground into

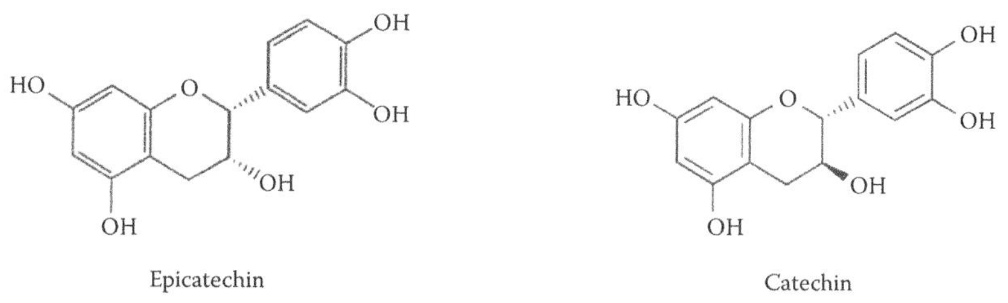

Epicatechin   Catechin

Figure 8.5 Active polyphenol molecules in chocolate.

a liquid form (known as chocolate liquor), which can be separated into cocoa solids (or powder) and cocoa butter. Chocolate is made by mixing different amounts of cocoa solids and cocoa butter with other ingredients such as sugar, milk, and flavoring. Although each of these steps degrades the flavanol content, an optional step called the Dutch process, in which cacao is treated with alkali to mellow its flavor, has a particular impact.[91] As a result, the cocoa or chocolate that we know of today is different from the cacao beverage consumed by traditional Mesoamerican cultures and has far less nutritional value.

Much of the fanfare associated with the medicinal benefits of chocolate originates from a few epidemiologic studies. The famous Seven Countries Study included an elderly population in the Dutch city Zutphen in which cocoa intake was found to be associated with lower blood pressure and a lower mortality rate from cardiovascular disease.[92] In another study of the indigenous Kuna Indians, who live in secluded islands off the coast of Panama, they were found to have a remarkably low rate of hypertension and cardiovascular disease despite consuming a relatively high-sodium diet. Tribesmen who migrated to the mainland did not share these health attributes. One of the differences between these two genetically similar groups is that the indigenous Kuna population consumed some 10-fold higher amounts of cocoa beverages compared with the migrated tribesmen.[93] More recent studies of chocolate consumption in both the United States and Sweden suggest protective effects from cardiovascular disease.[94,95] Despite these suggestive associations between chocolate and cardiovascular health, no controlled studies have confirmed this effect directly; most have focused on cardiovascular disease risk factors such as lipid levels, endothelial function, inflammatory markers, platelet adhesion properties, and blood pressure. Most studies show reduction in levels of total cholesterol and LDL cholesterol, and an increase in high-density lipoprotein (HDL) cholesterol.[96,97] Studies also show improved endothelial function with chocolate intake.[98,99] Favorable changes in inflammatory markers, such as reduced levels of oxidized LDL[100,101] and alteration of cytokine levels, such as increases in plasma prostacyclin and reduction in plasma leukotrienes,[102] also have been observed. Platelet adhesion, an important component of plaque development and atherosclerosis, is also attenuated.[103,104] Many studies measure the effect of chocolate on blood pressure, and although not uniformly agreed, a lowering effect has been observed in most. Typical reductions of 5/3 mm Hg[105,106] were seen in the general population, although a bigger effect may be seen in people with hypertension.[107] As suggested in several review articles, the main mechanism of blood pressure reduction is enhanced NO production with subsequent vasodilation.[108–110] However, inhibition of ACE also may contribute.[111] Chocolate consumption would therefore be predominantly a V-type method of lowering blood pressure, although an R- type component also may exist.

Although the benefits of chocolate are real, it is difficult to quantify the effects. This is partly due to a lack of standardized quantity and type of chocolate used in the studies. For example, quantities range from as little as 6 g a day to as much as 100 g. The type of chocolate—dark, milk, or cocoa powder—and the manufacturers of the products also differ between studies. As previously stated, processing has a large impact on the nutrient value, and the flavanol content may vary from as little as 200 mg to over 1000 mg. Unexpectedly, a dose effect was not observed as several of the lower-dose studies had better outcomes. These problems have a broader implication because of the lack of standardization in chocolate manufacturing. Many of the purported higher-end products advertise their cacao percentage, which is the percent by weight of cacao bean products within the chocolate. However, they are not obliged to further fractionate into the cocoa solid and cocoa butter components, which is most important from a medical viewpoint. For example, a 70% cacao chocolate bar may contain anywhere from 70% cocoa solids by weight and 0% cocoa butter to 0% cocoa solids and 70% cocoa butter. Because the cocoa solids contain the vital nutrients, it is impossible to compare the nutritional values of these products. To complicate matters further, other nutrients such as theobromine are found in cocoa and may also confer effect.[112] Furthermore, the frequency of chocolate consumption varies within the studies from only once daily intake to ingestion distributed throughout the day. This has relevance, as the plasma flavanol levels peak some 2 hours after consumption but are mostly gone after 6 hours.[113] Last, due to the cocoa butter component of chocolate, it is a high-caloric and fatty food that can be problematic for many people who suffer from cardiovascular disease and hypertension. The fat breakdown is about 60% from saturated fats (mostly stearic acid) and 40% from oleic acid, the monounsaturated fat found in olive oil. In its favor, stearic acid, despite being a saturated fat, has a relatively neutral effect on blood cholesterol levels,[114,115] although it still is highly caloric. Cocoa powder is a healthier alternative as it is mostly devoid of fat, is low in calories, and is rich in flavanol nutrients. Of importance is finding products that are relatively unprocessed, and although more expensive, higher-end cocoa powder from health food sites are a preferred choice. One such example is a product called CocoaVia produced by Mars Botanical, a division of Mars Incorporated (the maker of candy bars). They claim 350 mg of flavanols per serving of cocoa powder. They suggest adding it to other beverages such as coffee or milk probably as it has a bitter taste, although it certainly can be consumed as hot chocolate. Twice-daily servings at separate times should suffice and would offer comparable amounts of flavanols to most studies.

Tea

Tea is a commonly consumed beverage, second only to water in popularity. It originates from southeast Asia, and Chinese folklore claims its inception by the ancient emperor Shennong, who is also the father of traditional Chinese medicine. Legend tells of the emperor liking to drink boiled water when one day a leaf inadvertently landed in his pot to his surprised liking. Tea has a prominent role in traditional Chinese medicine and has gained a place in Western medicine as well. Most teas are made from the dried leaves of the plant camellia sinensis. They are notable for having high flavonoid content, specifically the catechins, a flavanol subgroup. Although somewhat confusing, catechins are a distinct group of compounds despite being structurally similar to the flavanol catechin found in cacao. In tea leaves, the important catechins are epigallocatechin gallate, epicatechin gallate, epicatechin, and epigallocatechin (Figure 8.6). Three variants of tea are commercially available—green, black, and oolong tea—which differ in processing. Green tea maintains the closest flavonoid composition to the natural leaf as it is first steamed or fired, inactivating a set of enzymes called polyphenol oxidases. These oxidases catalyze the oxidation of catechins into other flavanols called theaflavins and thearubigins. Green tea is then dried and crushed. Black tea is fermented prior to deactivation of the enzymes allowing oxidation to occur with concurrently lower amounts of catechins but higher amounts of theaflavins and thearubigins. Oolong tea is a hybrid, which is only partially fermented and contains intermediate levels of catechins, theaflavins, and thearubigins. Black

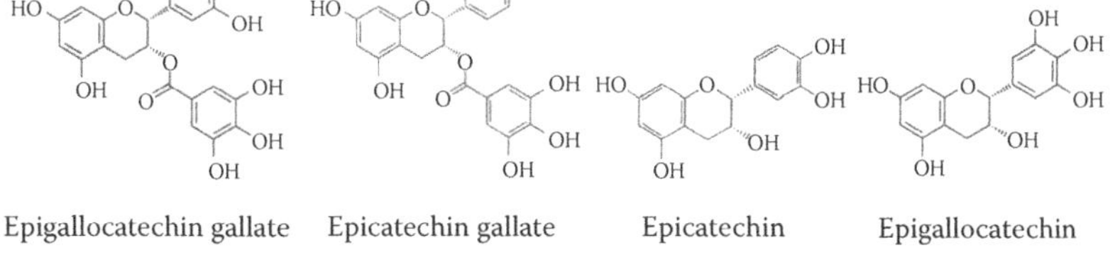

Epigallocatechin gallate   Epicatechin gallate   Epicatechin   Epigallocatechin

Figure 8.6 Active polyphenol molecules in tea.

tea is mostly popular in Europe and the United States, whereas green tea is more popular in Eastern Asia. This is important as studies from different parts of the world use different types of tea. The cardiovascular benefits of tea have been determined mostly from epidemiological studies. Large studies in Asia,[116,117] Europe,[118–120] and the United States[121,122] show an association of tea drinking with lower rates of cardiovascular disease. There are studies that suggest no association, particularly from the United Kingdom, but confounding socioeconomic factors and the habitual addition of milk to tea may explain these negative results.[123,124] A meta-analysis of people in Continental Europe (i.e., excluding the United Kingdom) confirms a positive association of tea consumption with protection from cardiovascular disease.[125] Incidence of stroke is also reduced.[126–128] Despite all of this supportive data, no definitive randomized controlled studies have been conducted to date. Similar to chocolate, most of the controlled studies involving tea have focused on cardiovascular disease risk factors rather than cardiovascular disease itself. However, these secondary attributes are not as clearly defined as those in chocolate, especially as most are from either animal studies or *in vitro* experiments.

The antioxidant ability of tea is perhaps its most important property and several studies confirm this effect by demonstrating improved antioxidant capacity[129,130] or reduced levels of oxidative markers such as lower levels of oxidized LDL[131–133] and lower C-reactive protein levels.[134] Studies also show improved lipid profiles,[135,136] although this has not been uniformly found.[137,138] Endothelial function is improved,[139–141] but this effect may not be a lasting one.[142] Platelet adhesion and platelet activity have been reduced in some studies[134,143] but not in others.[144] Protective effects against various malignancies such as breast,[145] prostate,[146,147] colorectal,[148] and lung cancer[149] also have been noted, probably due to its antioxidant properties. The effect of tea drinking on blood pressure is inconclusive. Although some studies show a blood-pressure-lowering effect, most do not.[106,150] In fact, tea may even cause an increase in blood pressure within 30 minutes of consumption.[151] There are, however, a few studies that suggest an antihypertensive effect in people with hypertension and in the elderly. One study using daily tea extract containing the equivalent of three to four cups of green tea suggests a reduction of systolic/diastolic blood pressure of 6/2 mm Hg.[152] Another study suggests a decrease of 2/1 mm Hg for every cup of green or black tea consumed daily.[153] However, overall the evidence for tea in lowering blood pressure is not clearly defined. Despite all these ambiguities, the ability of tea to attenuate cardiovascular disease and its risk factors is likely a real effect. The mechanisms involved are mostly attributable to antioxidant effects and the promotion of NO synthesis.[154,155] A small effect may arise from inhibition of ACE and the renin–angiotensin system (RAS).[156] Tea consumption would therefore be predominantly a V-type method of lowering blood pressure although an R-type component also may exist. Some of the difficulty in interpreting the data is, again, due to a lack of standardization in the studies making it difficult to compare one study with another. In addition, the flavonoid content of green tea differs from that of black tea. There is also variation in flavonoid content depending on the harvesting location, type of processing, and the form consumed (i.e., brewed or extract form).[157,158] Cup size, which can be as little as 90 mL or as much as 200 mL, and the number of cups consumed each day also vary within studies. Last, the bioavailability of the catechins (and presumably the theaflavins and thearubigins) is very low due to significant metabolism within the body[159] and the half-lives of these chemicals are only 2 to 5 hours.[160] Therefore, frequent and large amounts must be consumed to maintain a steady blood level. Given all these vagaries, it is difficult to recommend tea consumption at this time. Those who already drink tea regularly may continue, although the specific amount needed to confer benefit is not clear. Although green tea is often promoted as the healthier variant, this finding is not reflected in the scientific data. Green and black tea extracts are also commercially available in capsule form with each containing the flavonoid equivalent of several cups of tea. Some of these products specify the amount of catechins within.

Red wine (alcohol, resveratrol, and quercetin)

Wine consumption has societal importance and ancient origins. Although historically considered a luxury item—or perhaps even a vice—alcohol, and red wine in particular, has been associated more recently with improved health. The "French paradox" describes the finding of relatively low rates of cardiovascular disease in France despite unhealthy practices such as smoking and including saturated fats in the diet.[161] Regular consumption of red wine has been suggested as a contributing factor. To adequately explain the health effects of red wine, a description of its components, which include alcohol and various polyphenols, is needed. The following will first describe the effects of alcohol on health and hypertension and thereafter focus on red wine and its polyphenols.

There is considerable evidence that light to moderate alcohol consumption—up to 2 drinks per day in men and 1 in women—has beneficial health effects. An important source of confusion is the country-by-country variation in the quantity of alcohol within a standard drink, complicating the comparison of studies. In the United States, a standard drink contains 14 g of ethanol (pure alcohol), which is equivalent to either 1.5 fluid ounces (45 mL) of liquor (80 proof/40%), 5 fluid ounces (148 mL) of wine (12%), or 12 fluid ounces (355 mL) of beer (5%). As no conclusive prospective, randomized, controlled study of the health effects of alcohol has been done—nor is it likely ever to be performed—most of the data comes from epidemiological studies involving large populations and showing convincing effect. Many show a U- or J-shaped curve when comparing alcohol consumption with either overall mortality rate,[162,163] cardiovascular disease-associated mortality rate,[164–166] or cardiovascular disease incidence.[167] Such a curve describes results where the lowest rates of adverse events occur with light to moderate alcohol consumption compared with either total abstinence or heavy drinking. Several meta-analyses confirm these findings.[168,169] Protection from specific cardiovascular events such as sudden cardiac death[170] and myocardial infarction[171,172] importantly contribute to its effect. Attenuation of cardiovascular risk factors, as evidenced by increased HDL cholesterol levels,[166,169] improved endothelial function,[173] and improved markers of inflammation such as lower C-reactive protein levels[174] also have been shown. Surprisingly, the effect of alcohol consumption on stroke is unclear; there are conflicting data on protection from ischemic stroke, although heavy drinking has been associated with hemorrhagic stroke.[175] Despite its beneficial cardiovascular effects, alcohol is associated with increased blood pressure, and chronic drinking may contribute to as much as 10% of hypertension incidence.[176] Most studies show a progressive increase in blood pressure with alcohol intake,[177,178] although a few suggest possible lowering with one to three drinks each day.[179] The overall consensus is that alcohol directly causes blood pressure elevation,[180] although the effect resolves within weeks of cessation. Possible mechanisms include stimulation of the sympathetic nervous system[181] and the RAS.[182]

Wine can be broadly classified into two types, red and white, although there are many subtypes. Whether red wine provides more health benefit than white wine or other alcohol products is debated. The high polyphenol content of red wine is thought to confer an added benefit. Red wine differs from white wine in its processing, as the skins, seeds, and sometimes stems—which are a source of polyphenols—are allowed to ferment with the wine and impart color and nutrients. Unfortunately, no clear (randomized and controlled) studies have shown a superior effect of red wine, although many studies of lesser quality suggest this. An attempt to validate this claim can be approached by a three step process: (1) by first showing all wine types to have superior benefit to alcohol; (2) by showing that red wine is better than white wine; and (3) by evaluating the effects of dealcoholized red wine, purple grape juice, and red wine extract, which contain the nonalcohol components of red wine. Epidemiological studies and meta-analyses suggest that light to moderate wine consumption has superior benefit on all-cause mortality, cardiovascular disease mortality, and cardiovascular disease incidence, in comparison to other alcohol sources.[168,183,184] These studies combined include several hundred thousand participants, which is impressive and seemingly convincing. However, some think this is not conclusive evidence because socioeconomic factors such as diet, physical activity, obesity, and smoking habits differ between wine and other alcohol drinkers and may impart a confounding effect.[185-187] Some studies even suggest that wine has no benefit over other alcohol products,[188,189] although overall the data indicates a superior health benefit. That red wine is superior to white wine is suggested by studies showing attenuation of cardiovascular disease risk factors such as improved cholesterol levels, antioxidant effects,[190] and enhanced endothelial function,[191] although other studies fail to show a difference.[192] In summary, the initial argument that wine, and particularly red wine, is superior to alcohol is likely true, although it is not strongly supported. Because dealcoholized red wine, purple grape juice, and red wine extract also confer health benefits, there is a stronger argument that red wine polyphenols provide an extra effect in addition to that of alcohol alone. Unfortunately, most supporting data are from small studies on cardiovascular risk factors and not on cardiovascular disease itself. Evidence for improved endothelial function,[193,194] favorable antioxidant properties (particularly reduced LDL oxidation),[195-197] and inhibition of platelet aggregation[198,199] and of vascular smooth muscle cell proliferation[200] have been demonstrated. Correction of these risk factors is presumed to be protective of atherosclerosis and the development of cardiovascular disease, but they are still indirect markers. Several animal studies have shown an antihypertensive effect, mostly mediated by increased NO levels and presumed vasodilation.[201-203] A few small studies of people with hypertension also show a blood-pressure-lowering effect.[204-206] One study in men with hypertension reported a reduction of systolic/diastolic blood pressure of 4/3 mg Hg with consumption of about one cup of concord grape juice each day.[206] However, a study of healthy people without hypertension failed to show reduction in blood pressure with either dealcoholized red wine or red wine itself.[207] This nil effect is commonly observed in healthy individuals subjected to any type of antioxidant or endothelial-function-improving agent and is likely due to a lack of pathology in need of correction. Other studies in healthy people also have failed to show improvement in endothelial function[208] or other markers of inflammation[209] with red wine polyphenols. These compounds predominantly work by promoting NO production,[210,211] although they may also block the RAS by inhibiting ACE.[156,212]

Although there are several red wine polyphenols, only a few have received attention, as they likely confer most of the effect. Resveratrol, a nonflavonoid polyphenol belonging to the stilbene class, is likely the most efficacious although the flavonoids quercitin, catechin, and epicatechin are also important (Figure 8.7). Resveratrol is produced in the skin of grapes in response to noxious environmental stimuli, such as fungal infections, UV light exposure, and lack of water. Resveratrol is a natural antioxidant that protects the grapes from these elements. Not surprisingly, it also has anticarcinogenic effects.[213] As the focus on resveratrol is relatively new, few studies in animals or humans have been performed and most of the

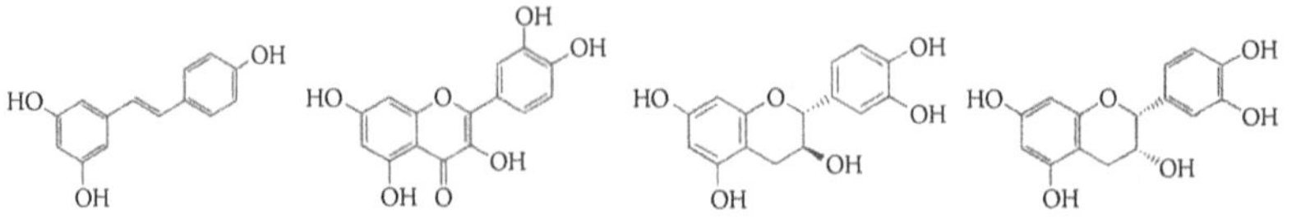

Figure 8.7 Active polyphenol molecules in red wine.

data is from *in vitro*/laboratory studies. Therefore, its claimed beneficial health effects are mostly derived from a presumed response rather than from direct measurement. Studies have suggested antioxidant effects,[214,215] anti-inflammatory effects,[216,217] inhibition of platelet aggregation,[218] and inhibition of vascular smooth muscle proliferation,[219] which all should minimize atherosclerosis and cardiovascular disease. Also reported is enhanced NO production,[220,221] which presumably improves endothelial function, and blockade of angiotensin II-mediated pathways.[222] Only a few studies in humans are available. One study in healthy individuals who took daily supplements of a plant extract containing 40 mg of resveratrol showed significantly improved parameters of systemic inflammation compared with a placebo group.[223] Another study involved obese women with hypertension who took daily doses of 30 to 270 mg and showed improved endothelial function.[224] The effect of resveratrol on blood pressure is not yet defined. A key point in assuming that these *in vitro* and *in vivo* studies of resveratrol can be extrapolated to human benefit with red wine consumption is whether a reasonable intake of red wine will allow the blood plasma level of resveratrol to reach a level comparable to those in the studies. Complicating these calculations, the polyphenol content of red wine varies by the type of wine, location of harvesting, and processing. For example, pinot noir from Australia has a significantly higher concentration of resveratrol than cabernet sauvignon from California.[225] Furthermore, the levels of free blood plasma resveratrol are relatively low, as most of the absorbed compound is in metabolized forms with undetermined effects.[226] One study showed that with inclusion of all forms of resveratrol, free nonmetabolized and metabolized, it is feasible that blood plasma levels can achieve an efficacious range with consumption of one half bottle of red wine a day,[225] although this is clearly speculative. Resveratrol extract is commercially available in moderate doses such as 20 and 40 mg tablets, which are equivalent to several liters of red wine, and in megadoses of 500 mg, which will likely yield significantly higher blood plasma levels. Although few reported side effects occur even with megadoses, there is not yet sufficient evidence to support the benefit of resveratrol supplementation on cardiovascular disease or hypertension. Last, and perhaps of most importance and of great excitement and potential, is a possible effect of resveratrol on activating a gene called Sirt1, which may help in life prolongation. Resveratrol is considered by some to be a fountain-of-youth elixir and this notion has attracted considerable attention, including that of major pharmaceutical companies. The Sirt1 gene regulates production of an enzyme called sirtuin 1, which controls cell cycle activity and glucose metabolism. Studies in various organisms, from yeasts to mammals, show that calorie deprivation and starvation is associated with a prolonged lifespan and improved insulin sensitivity. Activation of the Sirt1 gene is likely the causative factor.[227] Resveratrol has also been shown to prolong life and improve insulin sensitivity in mouse studies, likely via induction of this same gene.[228] However, the study doses used are quite high, although they can be provided with the megadose supplements, and no human studies are yet available. Needless to say, this would be a significant advancement in pharmacotherapy, if true. Some suggest 5 mg per kg of body weight is a reasonable dose comparable to the mouse study, whereas others suggest taking 500 mg daily. However, no clear data is currently available determining the proper dose or even whether its effect occurs in humans.

Far fewer studies have been performed on the effects of quercetin, a flavonoid, although these studies focus more directly on animal and human health as opposed to *in vitro* laboratory testing. Although there are no claims to life-extending properties, many studies suggest improvement in cardiovascular disease risk factors. Quercetin has been shown to improve endothelial function,[229,230] reduce systemic inflammation, improve insulin sensitivity, and improve lipid profiles.[231] *In vitro* laboratory studies show beneficial antioxidant properties with inhibition of LDL cholesterol oxidation[232] and vascular smooth muscle cell proliferation.[233] *In vivo* studies show antihypertensive effects.[234] A human study reports a reduction in systolic/diastolic blood pressure of 7/5 mm Hg in people with hypertension given 730 mg daily supplementation for 4 weeks, although there is no effect in prehypertensive people.[235] A study involving overweight individuals shows a reduction in systolic blood pressure of 3 mm Hg with daily supplementation of quercetin 150 mg for 5 weeks.[236] Possible mechanisms include increased NO production[229] and ACE inhibition.[237] Although promising in protecting from cardiovascular disease and lowering blood pressure, there is insufficient evidence to strongly recommend quercetin supplementation at this time.

Catechin and epicatechin are the final red wine polyphenols with purported effect. These flavonoids were discussed in the previous section on chocolate.

In summary, red wine appears to have protective properties against cardiovascular disease beyond those of alcohol alone. Its polyphenol content probably provides this added effect. Although red wine extract and its individual polyphenols are commercially available, there is not yet sufficient data to recommend their use. Despite its beneficial cardiovascular effects, it is also difficult to recommend red wine in those who are not already drinking regularly, as it may lead to addiction, overuse, and liver disease. For those already imbibing, the recommended amounts are up to 2 glasses a day for men and 1 glass for women.[175] However, there is no benefit of red wine in treating elevated blood pressure.

Taurine (2-aminoethanesulfonic acid)

Taurine is an important constituent of the diet with many health effects. Although often referred to as an amino acid, it is technically not, as it is a sulfonic acid rather than a carboxylic acid. Also, taurine is not a typical constituent of complex protein because it mostly exists in a free state within cellular cytoplasm or blood plasma. In humans, who have limited ability to synthesize it, it is mostly obtained through the diet. It was first discovered in 1827 as a component of ox bile, hence its name, but its importance was realized in the 1970s when formula-fed infants were found to be taurine-deficient and subsequently manifested developmental abnormalities.[238] Since then, it has been shown to be a vital component of cardiovascular health and blood pressure control in humans and other species. Several commercial energy drinks contain large amounts of taurine, claiming its importance in sustaining vitality and strength. Taurine supplementation, and conversely its deficiency, has been shown to have cardiovascular protective effects. This has been noted in a range of publications including randomized controlled human and animal studies, epidemiologic studies, and *in vitro*/laboratory studies. The WHO-CARDIAC study, undertaken to evaluate the role of nutrition in cardiovascular health, was a large, epidemiological, multicultural study including many populations from various countries. In its results, a relationship between taurine consumption and reduced cardiovascular disease mortality and stroke was shown.[239,240] Of particular distinction, the Japanese cohort, which had significantly lower rates of cardiovascular events, have very high taurine intake associated with their seafood-based diet.[241] Protection from aftereffects of cardiac ischemic events—known as ischemic reperfusion injury—that occur with coronary bypass surgery,[242] and improvement of cardiac contractility in states of heart failure[243–245] are also shown. Regulation of cellular calcium levels via modulation of cell-wall calcium and sodium channels is believed to be the mechanism conferring protection.[246–248] Cardiovascular disease risk factors are also positively affected by taurine consumption. Blood lipid profiles are improved, with reduced LDL cholesterol and triglyceride levels.[249–251] This is due to increased bile acid production in the liver via enhanced activity of the enzyme cholesterol-7-alpha-hydroxylase, which catalyzes the conversion of cholesterol to bile acid. Bile acid and cholesterol are subsequently eliminated from the body in the stool.[252] Taurine also upregulates hepatic cell LDL receptors causing reduced blood LDL cholesterol levels.[252] It also has an anti-inflammatory and antioxidant effect in part due to conjugation with hypochlorous acid (HOCl) forming taurine chloramine (Tau-Cl). Hypochlorous acid is produced by macrophages during inflammation such as during infection or with ischemic events such as myocardial infarction. Although its primary role is to oxidize infectious agents, it secondarily and inadvertently interacts with other tissue causing cell damage and necrosis.[253] When bound to taurine, hypochlorus acid is rendered less harmful.[254] Other risk factors are affected by taurine supplementation, for example, atherosclerosis is reduced or prevented,[255] endothelial dysfunction reversed,[256,257] platelet aggregation minimized,[258] and insulin sensitivity improved.[259] Blood pressure regulation is also closely related to taurine levels. An association exists between low levels in blood plasma and in urine and with essential hypertension.[260,261] Epidemiological studies also support a relationship between higher taurine intake and lower blood pressure.[262,263] A small study of young people with borderline hypertension, presumably essential hypertension, shows a reduction of systolic/diastolic blood pressure of 9/4 mm Hg with daily supplementation of 6 g of taurine.[264] However, most supporting data comes from animal models of hypertension, including salt-mediated hypertension,[265,266] renin-mediated hypertension,[267] and essential hypertension.[268,269] The mechanism by which taurine lowers blood pressure is likely multifactorial, including reduction in central nervous system sympathetic activity, blockade of the RAS, and increase in NO levels.[270] Catecholamine levels are significantly reduced,[268,271] as taurine has a probable central nervous system suppressant effect. This may be associated with increased endogenous opiate levels, and animal studies show a reduced sense of anxiety with taurine supplementation.[272,273] Blockade of the RAS may be from direct inhibition of angiotensin II[274] or from inhibition of ACE.[275] Kinin levels are increased, which may occur with ACE inhibition.[275] Taurine would therefore be a mixed V- and R-type method of lowering blood pressure.

The exact amount needed to confer effect is uncertain, as few human studies in hypertension or other diseases have been done. The range of supplementation in these studies varies from as little as 400 mg to 6 g daily.[246] The choice of taurine supplementation should ideally come from the diet and seafood is a good source. Table 8.1 provides a list of food sources of taurine. However, to approach the amounts used in these studies oral supplementation must also be considered, although this may be cumbersome, as a typical taurine tablet contains only 500 mg, which would require many tablets each day. Although supplementation of large amounts is considered relatively safe, side effects may occur with more than 3 g a day.[276] Yet, this also requires taking six pills a day, which is not reasonable. Despite the lack of strong scientific evidence, a recommendation of 1 g taken as 500 mg dose twice daily can be suggested. This dosage is based on epidemiological studies in which taurine was attained from

Table 8.1 Common Taurine-Rich Foods

Food item	Taurine content (mg/100 g)
Scallop, raw	823 mg
Mussels, raw	655 mg
Octopus, raw	388 mg
Squid, raw	357 mg
Clams, raw	240 mg
White fish, cooked	172 mg
Oysters, fresh	70 mg
Tuna, albacore, canned	42 mg
Cod, frozen	31 mg
Turkey dark meat, roasted	300 mg
Chicken dark meat, broiled	199 mg
Bologna turkey, cured	123 mg
Salami, cured	59 mg
Pork loin, roasted	57 mg
Veal, broiled	47 mg
Beef, broiled	38 mg

Source: Wójcik OP, Koenig KL, Zeleniuch-Jacquotte A, Costa M, Chen Y, The potential protective effects of taurine on coronary heart disease, *Atherosclerosis*, 2010;208:19–25.

food sources, and despite consumption of less than 1 g each day blood pressure was reduced and cardiovascular disease prevented.

Alpha-lipoic acid (1,2-dithiolane-3-pentanoic acid)

Alpha-lipoic acid (ALA) is a sulfur-based substance with many medicinal purposes. Its traditional and better-known function is as a cofactor to mitochondrial enzymes involved in aerobic respiration. However, when in its nonbound or free form, other functions have more recently been described. Naturally occurring ALA is bound to protein molecules and is obtained mostly through endogenous production as well as through diet. Foods such as muscle meats, spinach, broccoli, tomatoes, peas, and rice bran are good natural sources.[277] However, most commercial ALA supplements are synthetic products that are not protein bound (i.e., free form) and have different biologic effects. As most *in vivo* and *in vitro* studies use the synthetic formulation, it is difficult to extrapolate its effect when consumed in the natural form. Furthermore, the doses of synthetic ALA supplementation used in the studies are much higher than can be achieved by dietary intake. Therefore, ALA supplementation, although a holistic approach, may be considered more like a drug than a natural substance when taken in pill form. Further complicating matters, synthetic ALA is composed of two enantiomers, the R and L forms, which are stereoisomers or mirror images of each other, whereas naturally produced ALA is exclusively in the R form. From a chemical perspective, the two enantiomers have equal properties, but in biological terms they have different functions, as enzymes are very sensitive to chemical structure. Perhaps it is better to consider ALA a pharmaceutical agent.

ALA supplementation is regarded for its antioxidant effect and its ability to ameliorate diabetes control and diabetes-related illness. In human and animal cells, it is chemically reduced to dihydrolipoic acid (DHLA) by mitochondrial enzymes (Figure 8.8) and the pair have a redox potential of 0.32 eV, which is even greater than that of glutathione and its oxidized product. This makes it a very potent antioxidant with the ability to restore other antioxidants, such as glutathione, vitamin C, and indirectly vitamin E, to their active and reduced forms, as well as to quench reactive oxygen species.[278]

ALA also has unique hydrophilic and hydrophobic properties allowing it to exist and function in many biological compartments such as the cytoplasm, the cell wall, and the plasma. Supplementation has been shown to reduce systemic inflammation, reverse endothelial dysfunction,[279] improve cholesterol profiles, and reduce atherosclerosis.[280] Research into its effect on diabetes is promising as well. Several studies show improved insulin sensitivity,[281–283] likely mediated by redistribution of the glucose transporters, GLUT1 and GLUT4, from the cytoplasm to the cell wall, which facilitates glucose influx into cells.[284] Studies also show its effectiveness in treating diabetic peripheral neuropathy[285–288] and cardiac autonomic neuropathy.[289] There are a few studies, mostly in animal models, of the effect of ALA on blood pressure. Dietary supplementation in hypertensive rat models attenuates the onset of hypertension[290–293] and lowers blood pressure.[294] A small double-blind human study of ALA and carnitine supplementation in individuals with coronary artery disease showed a reduction in systolic blood pressure of 9 mm Hg in the hypertensive subgroup and 7 mm Hg in a metabolic syndrome subgroup after 4 weeks of treatment.[295] Possible mechanisms include reduced cytosolic calcium influx, reduced

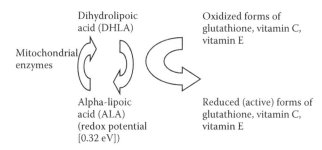

Figure 8.8 Mechanism of antioxidant effects of alpha-lipoic acid.

endothelin-1 production,[296] and enhanced NO synthesis. This would suggest a V-type method of lowering blood pressure, but the paucity of studies make it difficult to recommend its use in managing blood pressure. A sufficient dosage to achieve most cardiovascular, diabetic, and potential blood pressure goals would be 600 mg once daily. This dosage is based on several of the large studies, mostly in individuals with diabetes, which show significant beneficial effects without adverse side effects.[297]

A summary of the various supplements, suggested dosages, and common side effects are presented in Table 8.2.

Table 8.2 List of Dietary Supplements, Doses, and Side Effects

Dietary supplement	Dosages	Common side effects
L-arginine	3 tablets (350 mg each) sustained release twice daily	Increased mortality risk with recent myocardial infarct, airway inflammation, abdominal pain, bloating, diarrhea, gout
Coenzyme Q_{10}	100 mg daily	Elevated liver enzymes, wheezing, diarrhea, nausea
Garlic	Fresh raw garlic 4 g (1–2 cloves) daily Dried powder (1.3 percent alliin) 300 mg three times daily Aged garlic (7.2 g) daily	Increased bleeding risk, halitosis, facial swelling, eczema, diarrhea, nausea
Cocoa powder	One serving twice daily (use high-end unprocessed brand)	Anxiety, elevated blood glucose, irregular heart rate, headache, gastroesophageal reflux, diarrhea, constipation
Resveratrol	40 to 500 mg daily	Increased bleeding risk, insomnia, flu-like symptoms, diarrhea
Quercitin	250 to 750 mg daily (can be in divided dose twice daily)	Gastroesophageal reflux, wheezing, diarrhea, nausea, sweating
Taurine	500 mg twice daily	Increased bleeding, low blood glucose, mania, gastroesophageal reflux
Alpha-lipoic acid	600 mg once daily	Thyroid disease, low blood glucose, diarrhea, nausea, muscle cramps, fatigue
Red wine	Does not lower blood pressure	
Soy protein	Not practical in lowering blood pressure	
Tea and tea extract	Not recommended	

References

1. Sapa RB, Phillips RS, Sehgal A, et al. Lead, mercury, and arsenic in U.S.- and Indian-manufactured Ayurvedic medicines sold via the Internet. *JAMA*. 2008;300:915–923.

2. Wojcikowski K, Johnson DW, Gobe G. Medicinal herbal extracts—Renal friend or foe? Part one: The toxicities of medicinal herbs. *Nephrology (Carlton)*. 2004;9:313–318.

3. Buettner C, Mukamal KJ, Gardiner P, Davis RB, Phillips RS, Mittleman MA. Herbal supplement use and blood levels of United States adults. *J Gen Intern Med*. 2009;24:1175–1182.

4. Adams MR, Forsyth CJ, Jessup W, Robinson J, Celermajer DS. Oral L-arginine inhibits platelet aggregation but does not enhance endothelium-dependent dilation in healthy young men. *J Am Coll Cardiol*. 1995;26:1054–1061.

5. Blum A, Hathaway L, Mincemoyer R, et al. Effects of oral L-arginine on endothelium-dependent vasodilation and markers of inflammation in healthy postmenopausal women. *J Am Coll Cardiol*. 2000;35:271–276.

6. Chin-Dusting JP, Kaye DM, Lefkovits J, Wong J, Bergin P, Jennings GL. Dietary supplementation with L-arginine fails to restore endothelial function in forearm resistance arteries of patients with severe heart failure. *J Am Coll Cardiol*. 1996;27:1207–1213.

7. Schulman SP, Becker LC, Kass DA, et al. L-arginine therapy in acute myocardial infarction: The Vascular Interaction With Age in Myocardial Infarction (VINTAGE MI) randomized clinical trial. *JAMA*. 2006;295:58–64.

8. Clarkson P, Adams MR, Powe AJ, et al. Oral L-arginine improves endothelium-dependent dilation of hypercholesterolemic young adults. *J Clin Invest*. 1996;97:1989–1994.

9. Adams MR, McCredie R, Jessup W, Robinson J, Sullivan D, Celermajer DS. Oral L-arginine improves endothelium-dependent dilation and reduces monocyte adhesion to endothelial cells in young men with coronary artery disease. *Atherosclerosis*. 1997;129:261–269.

10. Hambrecht R, Hilbrich L, Erbs S, et al. Correction of endothelial dysfunction in chronic heart failure: Additional effects of exercise training and oral L-arginine supplementation. *J Am Coll Cardiol*. 2000;35:706–713.

11. Bode-Böger SM, Muke J, Surdacki A, Brabant G, Böger RH, Frölich JC. Oral L-arginine improves endothelial function in healthy individuals older than 70 years. *Vasc Med*. 2003;8:77–81.

12. Böger RH. Asymmetric dimethylarginine, an endogenous inhibitor of nitric oxide synthase, explains the "L-arginine paradox" and acts as a novel cardiovascular risk factor. *J Nutr*. 2004;134(10 suppl):2842S–2847S.

13. Böger RH, Bode-Böger SM, Szuba A, et al. Asymmetric dimethylarginine (ADMA): A novel risk factor for endothelial dysfunction. Its role in hypercholesterolemia. *Circulation*. 1998;98:1842–1847.

14. Bode-Böger SM, Scalera F, Ignarro LJ. The L-arginine paradox: Importance of the L-arginine/asymmetrical dimethylarginine ratio. *Pharmacol Ther*. 2007;114:295–306.

15. Loscalzo J. L-arginine and atherothrombosis. *J Nutr*. 2004;134(10 suppl): 2799S–2800S.

16. Siani A, Pagano E, Iacone R, Iacoviello L, Scopacasa F, Strazzullo P. Blood pressure and metabolic changes during dietary L-arginine supplementation in humans. *Am J Hypertens.* 2000;13(5 Pt 1):547–551.
17. Miller AL. The effects of a sustained-release L-arginine formulation on blood pressure and vascular compliance in 29 healthy individuals. *Altern Med Rev.* 2006;11:23–29.
18. Higashi Y, Oshima T, Ozono R, Watanabe M, Matsuura H, Kajiyama G. Effects of L-arginine infusion on renal hemodynamics in patients with mild essential hypertension. *Hypertension.* 1995;25(4 Pt 2):898–902.
19. Mehta S, Stewart DJ, Levy RD. The hypotensive effect of L-arginine is associated with increased expired nitric oxide in humans. *Chest.* 1996;109:1550–1555.
20. Wilcox CS, Welch WJ, Murad F, et al. Nitric oxide synthase in macula densa regulates glomerular capillary pressure. *Proc Natl Acad Sci USA.* 1992;89:11993–1197.
21. Shultz PJ, Tolins JP. Adaptation to increased dietary salt intake in the rat. *J Clin Invest.* 1993;91:642–650.
22. Higashi Y, Oshima T, Ono N, et al. Intravenous administration of L-arginine inhibits angiotensin-converting enzyme in humans. *J Clin Endocrinol Metab.* 1995;80:2198–2202.
23. Kurtz A, Wagner C. Role of nitric oxide in the control of renin secretion. *Am J Physiol.* 1998;275(6 Pt 2):F849–F862.
24. Pedrinelli R, Ebel M, Catapano G, et al. Pressor, renal and endocrine effects of L-arginine in essential hypertensives. *Eur J Clin Pharmacol.* 1995;48:195–201.
25. Hishikawa K, Nakaki T, Suzuki H, Kato R, Saruta T. Role of L-arginine-nitric oxide pathway in hypertension. *J Hypertens.* 1993;11:639–645.
26. Jula A, Marniemi J, Huupponen R, Virtanen A, Rastas M, Rönnemaa T. Effects of diet and Simvastatin on serum lipids, insulin, and antioxidants in hypercholesterolemic men: A randomized controlled trial. *JAMA.* 2002;287:598–605.
27. Ghirlanda G, Oradei A, Manto A, et al. Evidence of plasma CoQ_{10}-lowering effect by HMG-CoA reductase inhibitors: A double-blind, placebo-controlled study. *J Clin Pharmacol.* 1993;33:226–229.
28. Bleske BE, Willis RA, Anthony M, et al. The effect of pravastatin and artovastatin on coenzyme Q_{10}. *Am Heart J.* 2001;142:E2.
29. Kalén A, Appelkvist EL, Dallner G. Age-related changes in the lipid compositions of rat and human tissues. *Lipids.* 1989;24:579–584.
30. Shindo Y, Witt E, Han D, Packer L. Dose-response effects of acute ultraviolet irradiation on antioxidants and molecular markers of oxidation in murine epidermis and dermis. *J Invest Dermatol.* 1994;102:470–475.
31. Mortensen SA, Vadhanavikit S, Muratsu K, Folkers K. Coenzyme Q_{10}: Clinical benefits with biochemical correlates suggesting a scientific breakthrough in management of chronic heart failure. *Int J Tissue React.* 1990;12:155–162.
32. Baggio E, Gandini R, Plancher AC, Passeri M, Carmosino G. Italian multicenter study on the safety and efficiency of coenzyme Q_{10} as adjunctive therapy in heart failure. *Mol Aspects Med.* 1994; 15(suppl 1):S287–S294.
33. Morisco C, Trimarco B, Condorelli M. Effect of coenzyme Q_{10} therapy in patients with congestive heart failure: A long-term multicenter randomized study. *Clin Investig.* 1993; 71(8 suppl): S134–S136.

34. Soja AM, Mortensen SA. Treatment of congestive heart failure with coenzyme Q_{10} illuminated by meta-analyses of clinical trials. *Mol Aspects Med.* 1997; 18(suppl 1):S159–S168.
35. Khatta M, Alexander BS, Krichten CM, et al. The effect of coenzyme Q_{10} in patients with congestive heart failure. *Ann Intern Med.* 2000;132:636–640.
36. Watson PS, Scalia GM, Galbraith A, Burstow DJ, Bett N, Aroney CN. Lack of effect of coenzyme Q on left ventricular function in patients with congestive heart failure. *J Am Coll Cardiol.* 1999;33:1549–1552.
37. Tran MT, Mitchell TM, Kennedy DT, Giles JT. Role of coenzyme Q_{10} in chronic heart failure, angina, and hypertension. *Pharmacotherapy.* 2001;21:797–806.
38. Singh RB, Neki NS, Kartikey K, et al. Effect of coenzyme Q_{10} on risk of atherosclerosis in patients with recent myocardial infarction. *Mol Cell Biochem.* 2003;246:75–82.
39. Yamagami T, Shibata N, Folkers K. Bioenergetics in clinical medicine. Studies on coenzyme Q_{10} and essential hypertension. *Res Commun Chem Pathol Pharmacol.* 1975;11:273–288.
40. Ho MJ, Bellusci A, Wright JM. Blood pressure lowering efficacy of coenzyme Q_{10} for primary hypertension. *Cochrane Database Syst Rev.* 2009;7:CD007435.
41. Rosenfeldt FL, Haas SJ, Krum H, et al. Coenzyme Q_{10} in treatment of hypertension: A meta-analysis of the clinical trials. *J Hum Hypertens.* 2007;21:297–306.
42. Hodgson JM, Watts GF, Playford DA, Burke V, Croft KD. Coenzyme Q_{10} improves blood pressure and glycaemic control: A controlled trial in subjects with type 2 diabetes. *Eur J Clin Nutr.* 2002;56:1137–1142.
43. Shults CW, Oakes D, Kieburtz K, et al. Effects of coenzyme Q_{10} in early Parkinson disease: Evidence of slowing of the functional decline. *Arch Neurol.* 2002;59:1541–1550.
44. Sándor PS, Di Clemente L, Coppola G, et al. Efficacy of coenzyme Q_{10} in migraine prophylaxis: A randomized controlled trial. *Neurology.* 2005;64:713–715.
45. Lockwood K, Moesgaard S, Yamamoto T, Folkers K. Progress on therapy of breast cancer with vitamin Q_{10} and the regression of metastases. *Biochem Biphys Res Commun.* 1995;212:172–177.
46. Digiesi V, Cantini F, Oradei A, et al. Coenzyme Q_{10} in essential hypertension. *Mol Aspects Med.* 1994; 15(suppl 1):S257–S263.
47. Bonakdar RA, Guarneri E. Coenzyme Q_{10}. *Am Fam Physician.* 2005;72:1065–1070.
48. Landbo C, Almdal TP. Interaction between warfarin and coenzyme Q_{10}. *Ugeskr Laeger.* 1998;160:3226–3227.
49. Chopra RK, Goldman R, Sinatra ST, Bhagavan HN. Relative bioavailability of coenzyme Q_{10} formulations in human subjects. *Int J Vitam Nutr Res.* 1998;68:109–113.
50. Pravst I, Zmitek K, Zmitek J. Coenzyme Q_{10} contents in foods and fortification strategies. *Crit Rev Food Sci Nutr.* 2010;50:269–280.
51. Tattelman E. Health effects of garlic. *Am Fam Physician.* 2005;72:103–106.
52. Rahman K, Lowe GM. Garlic and cardiovascular disease: A critical review. *J Nutr.* 2006;136;(3 suppl):736S–740S.
53. Banerjee SK, Maulik SK. Effects of garlic on cardiovascular disorders: A review. *Nutr J.* 2002;1:4.

54. Budoff M. Aged garlic extract retards progression of coronary artery calcification. *J Nutr.* 2006;136(3 suppl):741S–744S.

55. Koscielny J, Klüssendorf D, Latza R, et al. The antiatherosclerotic effect of *Allium sativum. Atherosclerosis.* 1999;144:237–249.

56. Fleischauer AT, Arab L. Garlic and cancer: A critical review of the epidemiologic literature. *J Nutr.* 2001;131:1032S–1040S.

57. Fleischauer AT, Poole C, Arab L. Garlic consumption and cancer prevention: Meta-analysis of colorectal and stomach cancers. *Am J Clin Nutr.* 2000;72:1047–1052.

58. Josling P. Preventing the common cold with a garlic supplement: A double-blind, placebo-controlled survey. *Adv Ther.* 2001;18:189–193.

59. Reinhart KM, Coleman CI, Teevan C, Vachhani P, White CM. Effects of garlic on blood pressure in patients with and without systolic hypertension: A meta-analysis. *Ann Pharmacother.* 2008;42:1766–1771.

60. Ried K, Frank OR, Stocks NP, Fakler P, Sullivan T. Effect of garlic on blood pressure: A systematic review and meta-analysis. *BMC Cardiovasc Disord.* 2008;8:13.

61. Simons S, Wollersheim H, Thien T. A systematic review on the influence of trial quality on the effect of garlic on blood pressure. *Neth J Med.* 2009;67:212–219.

62. Mulrow C, Lawrence V, Ackermann R, et al. Garlic: Effects on cardiovascular risks and disease, protective effects against cancer, and clinical adverse effects. *Evid Rep Technol Assess (Summ).* 2000;20:1–4.

63. Sendl A, Elbl G, Steinke B, Redl K, Breu W, Wagner H. Comparative pharmacological investigations of *Allium ursinum* and *Allium sativum. Planta Med.* 1992;58:1–7.

64. Pedraza-Chaverri J, Tapia E, Medina-Campos ON, de los Angeles Granados M, Franco M. Garlic prevents hypertension induced by chronic inhibition of nitric oxide synthesis. *Life Sci.* 1998;62:71–77.

65. Das I, Tapia E, Medina-Campos ON, de los Angeles Granados M, Franco M. Potent activation of nitric oxide synthase by garlic: A basis for its therapeutic applications. *Curr Med Res Opin.* 1995;13:257–263.

66. Kaye AD, De Witt BJ, Anwar M, et al. Analysis of responses of garlic derivatives in the pulmonary vascular bed of the rat. *J Appl Physiol.* 2000;89:353–358.

67. Manach C, Scalbert A, Morand C, Rémésy C, Jiménez L. Polyphenols: Food sources and bioavailability. *Am J Clin Nutr.* 2004;79:727–747.

68. Hertog MG, Feskens EJ, Hollman PC, Katan MB, Kromhout D. Dietary antioxidant flavonoids and risk of coronary heart disease: The Zutphen Elderly Study. *Lancet.* 1993;342:1007–1011.

69. Geleijnse JM, Launer LJ, Van der Kuip DA, Hofman A, Witteman JC. Inverse association of tea and flavonoid intakes with incident myocardial infarction: The Rotterdam Study. *Am J Clin Nutr.* 2002;75:880–886.

70. Huxley RR, Neil HA. The relation between dietary flavonol intake and coronary heart disease mortality: A meta-analysis of prospective cohort studies. *Eur J Clin Nutr.* 2003;57:904–908.

71. Keli SO, Hertog MG, Feskens EJ, Kromhout D. Dietary flavonoids, antioxidant vitamins, and incidence of stroke: The Zutphen Elderly study. *Arch Intern Med.* 1996;156:637–642.

72. Anderson JW, Johnstone BM, Cook-Newell ME. Meta-analysis of the effects of soy protein intake on serum lipids. *N Engl J Med.* 1995;333:276–282.

73. Reynolds K, Chin A, Lees KA, Nguyen A, Bujnowski D, He J. A meta-analysis of the effect of soy protein supplementation on serum lipids. *Am J Cardiol.* 2006;98:633–640.

74. Taku K, Umegaki K, Sato Y, Taki Y, Endoh K, Watanabe S. Soy isoflavones lower serum total and LDL cholesterol in humans: A meta-analysis of 11 randomized controlled trials. *Am J Clin Nutr.* 2007;85:1148–1156.

75. Weggemans RM, Trautwein EA. Relation between soy-associated isoflavones and LDL and HDL cholesterol concentrations in humans: A meta-analysis. *Eur J Clin Nutr.* 2003;57:940–946.

76. Dewell A, Hollenbeck PL, Hollenbeck CB. Clinical review: A critical evaluation of the role of soy protein and isoflavone supplementation in the control of plasma cholesterol concentrations. *J Clin Endocrinol Metab.* 2006;91:772–780.

77. Sacks FM, Lichtenstein A, Van Horn L, Harris W, Kris-Etherton P, Winston M. Soy protein, isoflavones, and cardiovascular health: An American Heart Association Science Advisory for professionals from the Nutrition Committee. *Circulation.* 2006;113:1034–1044.

78. Tikkanen MJ, Wähälä K, Ojala S, Vihma V, Adlercreutz H. Effect of soybean phytoestrogen intake on low density lipoprotein oxidation resistance. *Proc Natl Acad Sci USA.* 1998;95:3106–3110.

79. Williams JK, Clarkson TB. Dietary soy isoflavones inhibit *in-vivo* constrictor responses of coronary arteries to collagen-induced platelet activation. *Coron Artery Dis.* 1998;9:759–764.

80. Anthony MS, Clarkson TB, Bullock BC, Wagner JD. Soy protein versus soy phytoestrogens in the prevention of diet-induced coronary artery atherosclerosis of male cynomolgus monkeys. *Arterioscler Thromb Vasc Biol.* 1997;17:2524–2531.

81. Trock BJ, Hilakivi-Clarke L, Clarke R. Meta-analysis of soy intake and breast cancer risk. *J Natl Cancer Inst.* 2006;98:459–471.

82. Albertazzi P, Pansini F, Bonaccorsi G, Zanotti L, Forini E, De Aloysio D. The effect of dietary soy supplementation on hot flushes. *Obstet Gynecol.* 1998;91:6–11.

83. Rivas M, Garay RP, Escanero JF, Cia P Jr, Cia P, Alda JO. Soy milk lowers blood pressure in men and women with mild to moderate essential hypertension. *J Nutr.* 2002;132:1900–1902.

84. He J, Gu D, Wu X, et al. Effect of soybean protein on blood pressure: A randomized, controlled trial. *Ann Intern Med.* 2005;143:1–9.

85. Teede HJ, Giannopoulos D, Dalais FS, Hodgson J, McGrath BP. Randomized, controlled, cross-over trial of soy protein with isoflavones on blood pressure and arterial function in hypertensive subjects. *J Am Coll Nutr.* 2006;25:533–540.

86. Hooper L, Kroon PA, Rimm EB, et al. Flavonoids, flavonoid-rich foods, and cardiovascular risk: A meta-analysis of randomized controlled trials. *Am J Clin Nutr.* 2008;88:38–50.

87. Yang HY, Chen JR, Chang LS. Effects of soy protein hydrolysate on blood pressure and angiotensin-converting enzyme activity in rats with chronic renal failure. *Hypertens Res.* 2008;31:957–963.

88. Martínez RM, Giménez I, Lou JM, Mayoral JA, Alda JO. Soy isoflavonoids exhibit *in vitro* biological activities of loop diuretics. *Am J Clin Nutr.* 1998;68(6 suppl):1354S–1357S.

89. Azadbakht L, Kimiagar M, Mehrabi Y, Esmaillzadeh A, Hu FB, Willett WC. Soy consumption, markers of inflammation, and endothelial function: A cross-over study in postmenopausal women with metabolic syndrome. *Diabetes Care.* 2007;30:967–973.

90. Henderson JS, Joyce RA, Hall GR, Hurst WJ, McGovern PE. Chemical and archeological evidence for the earliest cacao beverages. *Proc Natl Acad Sci USA.* 2007;104:18937–18940.

91. Payne MJ, Hurst WJ, Miller KB, Rank C, Stuart DA. Impact of fermentation, drying, roasting, and Dutch processing on epicatechin and catechin content of cacao beans and cocoa ingredients. *J Agric Food Chem.* 2010;58:10518–10527.

92. Buijsse B, Feskens EJ, Kok FJ, Kromhout D. Cocoa intake, blood pressure, and cardiovascular mortality: The Zutphen Elderly Study. *Arch Intern Med.* 2006;166:411–417.

93. McCullough ML, Chevaux K, Jackson L, et al. Hypertension, the Kuna, and the epidemiology of flavanols. *J Cardiovasc Pharmacol.* 2006;47(suppl 2):S103–S109.

94. Djoussé L, Hopkins PN, North KE, Pankow JS, Arnett DK, Ellison RC. Chocolate consumption is inversely associated with prevalent coronary heart disease: The National Heart, Lung, and Blood Institute Family Heart Study. *Clin Nutr.* 2011;30:182–187.

95. Mostofsky E, Levitan EB, Wolk A, Mittleman MA. Chocolate intake and incidence of heart failure: A population-based prospective study of middle-aged and elderly women. *Circ Heart Fail.* 2010;3:612–616.

96. Jia L, Liu X, Bai YY, et al. Short-term effect of cocoa product consumption on lipid profile: A meta-analysis of randomized controlled trials. *Am J Clin Nutr.* 2010;92:218–225.

97. Baba S, Natsume M, Yasuda A, et al. Plasma LDL and HDL cholesterol and oxidized LDL concentrations are in normo- and hypercholesterolemic humans after intake of different levels of cocoa powder. *J Nutr.* 2007;137:1436–1441.

98. Faridi Z, Njike VY, Dutta S, Ali A, Katz DL. Acute dark chocolate and cocoa ingestion and endothelial function: A randomized controlled crossover trial. *Am J Clin Nutr.* 2008;88:58–63.

99. Engler MB, Engler MM, Chen CY, et al. Flavonoid-rich dark chocolate improves endothelial function and increases plasma epicatechin concentrations in healthy adults. *J Am Coll Nutr.* 2004;23:197–204.

100. Kondo K, Hirano R, Matsumoto A, Igarashi O, Itakura H. Inhibition of LDL oxidation by cocoa. *Lancet.* 1996;348:1514.

101. Mathur S, Devaraj S, Grundy SM, Jialal I. Cocoa products decrease low density lipoprotein oxidative susceptibility but do not affect biomarkers of inflammation in humans. *J Nutr.* 2002;132:3663–3667.

102. Schramm DD, Wang JF, Holt RR, et al. Chocolate procyanidins decrease the leukotriene-prostacyclin ratio in humans and human aortic endothelial cells. *Am J Clin Nutr.* 2001;73:36–40.

103. Flammer AJ, Hermann F, Sudano I, et al. Dark chocolate improves coronary vasomotion and reduces platelet reactivity. *Circulation.* 2007;116:2376–2382.

104. Murphy KJ, Chronopoulos AK, Singh I, et al. Dietary flavanols and procyanidin oligomers from cocoa (*Theobroma cacao*) inhibit platelet function. *Am J Clin Nutr.* 2003;77:1466–1473.

105. Desch S, Schmidt J, Kobler D, et al. Effect of cocoa products on blood pressure: Systematic review and meta-analysis. *Am J Hypertens.* 2010;23:97–103.

106. Taubert D, Roesen R, Schömig E. Effect of cocoa and tea intake on blood pressure: A meta-analysis. *Arch Intern Med.* 2007;167:626–634.
107. Ried K, Sullivan T, Fakler P, Frank OR, Stocks NP. Does chocolate reduce blood pressure? A meta-analysis. *BMC Med.* 2010;8:39.
108. Corti R, Flammer AJ, Hollenberg NK, Lüscher TF. Cocoa and cardiovascular health. *Circulation.* 2009;119:1433–1441.
109. Engler MB, Engler MM. The emerging role of flavonoid-rich cocoa and chocolate in cardiovascular health and disease. *Nutr Rev.* 2006;64:109–118.
110. Fisher ND, Hughes M, Gerhard-Herman M, Hollenberg NK. Flavanol-rich cocoa induces nitric-oxide-dependent vasodilation in healthy humans. *J Hypertens.* 2003;21:2281–2286.
111. Persson IA, Persson K, Hägg S, Andersson RG. Effects of cocoa extract and dark chocolate on angiotensin-converting enzyme and nitric oxide in human endothelial cells and healthy volunteers—A nutrigenomics perspective. *J Cardiovasc Pharmacol.* 2011;57:44–50.
112. Kelly CJ. Effects of theobromine should be considered in future studies. *Am J Clin Nutr.* 2005;8:486–487.
113. Rein D, Lotito S, Holt RR, Keen CL, Schmitz HH, Fraga CG. Epicatechin in human plasma: *In vivo* determination and effect of chocolate consumption on plasma oxidation status. *J Nutr.* 2000;130(8S suppl):2109S–2114S.
114. Bonanome A, Grundy SM. Effect of dietary stearic acid on plasma cholesterol and lipoprotein levels. *N Engl J Med.* 1998;318:1244–1248.
115. Mensink RP, Zock PL, Kester AD, Katan MB. Effects of dietary fatty acids and carbohydrates on the ratio of serum total HDL cholesterol and on serum lipids and apolipoproteins: A meta-analysis of 60 controlled trials. *Am J Clin Nutr.* 2003;77:1146–1155.
116. Kuriyama S, Shimazu T, Ohmori K, et al. Green tea consumption and mortality due to cardiovascular disease, cancer and all causes in Japan: The Ohsaki study. *JAMA.* 2006;296:1255–1265.
117. Suzuki E, Yorifuji T, Takao S, et al. Green tea consumption and mortality among Japanese elderly people: The prospective Shizuoka elderly cohort. *Ann Epidemiol.* 2009;19:732–739.
118. de Koning Gans JM, Uiterwaal CS, van der Schouw YT, et al. Tea and coffee consumption and cardiovascular morbidity and mortality. *Arterioscler Thromb Vasc Biol.* 2010;30:1665–1671.
119. Geleijnse JM, Launer LJ, Hofman A, Pols HA, Witteman JC. Tea flavonoids may protect against atherosclerosis: The Rotterdam Study. *Arch Intern Med.* 1999;159:2170–2174.
120. Hertog MG, Feskens EJ, Hollman PC, Katan MB, Kromhout D. Dietary antioxidant flavonoids and risk of coronary heart disease: The Zutphen Elderly Study. *Lancet.* 1993;342:1007–1011.
121. Sesso HD, Gaziano JM, Buring JE, Hennekens CH. Coffee and tea intake and the risk of myocardial infarction. *Am J Epidemiol.* 1999;149:162–167.
122. Mukamal KJ, Maclure M, Muller JE, Sherwood JB, Mittleman MA. Tea consumption and mortality after acute myocardial infarction. *Circulation.* 2002;105:2476–2481.
123. Woodward M, Tunstall-Pedoe H. Coffee tea consumption in the Scottish Heart Health Study follow-up: Conflicting relations with coronary risk factors, coronary disease, and all cause mortality. *J Epidemiol Community Health.* 1999;53:481–487.

124. Hertog MG, Sweetnam PM, Fehily AM, Elwood PC, Kromhout D. Antioxidant flavonols and ischemic heart disease in a Welsh population of men: The Caerphilly Study. *Am J Clin Nutr.* 1997;65:1489–1494.

125. Peters U, Poole C, Arab L. Does tea affect cardiovascular disease? A meta-analysis. *Am J Epidemiol.* 2001;154:495–503.

126. Arab L, Liu W, Elashoff D. Green and black tea consumption and risk of stroke: A meta-analysis. *Stroke.* 2009;40:1786–1792.

127. Liang W, Lee AH, Binns CW, Huang R, Hu D, Zhou Q. Tea consumption and ischemic stroke risk: A case-control study in southern China. *Stroke.* 2009;40:2480–2485.

128. Tanabe N, Suzuki H, Aizawa Y, Seki N. Consumption of green and roasted teas and the risk of stroke incidence: Results from the Tokamachi-Nakasato cohort study in Japan. *Int J Epidemiol.* 2008;37:1030–1040.

129. Rietveld A, Wiseman S. Antioxidant effects of tea: Evidence from human clinical trials. *J Nutr.* 2003;133:3285S–3292S.

130. Leenen R, Roodenburg AJ, Tijburg LB, Wiseman SA. A single dose of tea with or without milk increases plasma antioxidant activity in humans. *Eur J Clin Nutr.* 2000;54:87–92.

131. Tinahones FJ, Rubio MA, Garrido-Sánchez L, et al. Green tea reduces LDL oxidability and improves vascular function. *J Am Coll Nutr.* 2008;27:209–213.

132. Inami S, Takano M, Yamamoto M, et al. Tea catechin consumption reduces circulating oxidized low-density lipoprotein. *Int Heart J.* 2007;48:725–732.

133. Lee W, Min WK, Chun S, et al. Long-term effects of green tea ingestion on atherosclerotic biological markers in smokers. *Clin Biochem.* 2005;38:84–87.

134. Steptoe A, Gibson EL, Vuononvirta R, et al. The effects of chronic tea intake on platelet activation and inflammation: A double-blind placebo controlled trial. *Atherosclerosis.* 2007;193:277–282.

135. Maron DJ, Lu GP, Cai NS, et al. Cholesterol-lowering effect of a theaflavin-enriched green tea extract: A randomized controlled trial. *Arch Intern Med.* 2003;163:1448–1453.

136. Imai K, Nakachi K. Cross-sectional study of effects of drinking green tea on cardiovascular and liver diseases. *BMJ.* 1995;310:693–696.

137. Mukamal KJ, MacDermott K, Vinson JA, Oyama N, Manning WJ, Mittleman MA. A 6-month randomized pilot study of black tea and cardiovascular risk factors. *Am Heart J.* 2007;154:724.e1-6.

138. Tsubono Y, Tsugane S. Green tea intake in relation to serum lipid levels in middle-aged Japanese men and women. *Ann Epidemiol.* 1997;7:280–284.

139. Grassi D, Mulder TP, Draijer R, Desideri G, Molhuizen HO, Ferri C. Black tea consumption dose-dependently improves flow mediated dilation in healthy males. *J Hypertens.* 2009;27:774–781.

140. Duffy SJ, Keaney JF Jr, Holbrook M, et al. Short-and long-term black tea consumption reverses endothelial dysfunction in patients with coronary artery disease. *Circulation.* 2001;104:151–156.

141. Moore RJ, Jackson KG, Minihane AM. Green tea (*Camellia sinensis*) catechins and vascular function. *Br J Nutr.* 2009;102:1790–1802.

142. Widlansky ME, Hamburg NM, Anter E, et al. Acute EGCG supplementation reverses endothelial dysfunction in patients with coronary artery disease. *J Am Coll Nutr.* 2007;26:95–102.

143. Kang WS, Lim IH, Yuk DY, et al. Antithrombotic activities of green tea catechins and (-)-epigallocatechin gallate. *Thromb Res.* 1999;96:229–237.

144. Duffy S, Vita JA, Holbrook M, Swerdloff PL, Keaney JF Jr. Effect of acute and chronic tea consumption on platelet aggregation in patients with coronary artery disease. *Arterioscler Thromb Vasc Biol.* 2001;21:1084–1089.
145. Sun CL, Yuan JM, Koh WP, Yu MC. Green tea, black tea and breast cancer risk: A meta-analysis of epidemiological studies. *Carcinogenesis.* 2006;27:1310–1315.
146. Kurahashi N, Sasazuki S, Iwasaki M, Inoue M, Tsugane S, JPHC Study Group. Green tea consumption and prostate cancer risk in Japanese men: A prospective study. *Am J Epidemiol.* 2008;167:71–77.
147. Bettuzzi S, Brausi M, Rizzi F, Castagnetti G, Peracchia G, Corti A. Chemoprevention of human prostate cancer by oral administration of green tea catechins in volunteers with high-grade prostate intraepithelial neoplasia: A preliminary report from a one-year proof-of-principle study. *Cancer Res.* 2006;66:1234–1240.
148. Sun CL, Yuan JM, Koh WP, Yu MC. Green tea, black tea and colorectal cancer risk: A meta-analysis of epidemiologic studies. *Carcinogenesis.* 2006;27:1301–1309.
149. Arts IC. A review of the epidemiological evidence on tea, flavonoids, and lung cancer. *J Nutr.* 2008;138:1561S–1566S.
150. Bingham SA, Vorster H, Jerling JC, et al. Effect of black tea drinking on blood lipids, blood pressure and aspects of bowel habit. *Br J Nutr.* 1997;78:41–55.
151. Hodgson JM, Puddey IB, Burke V, Beilin LJ, Jordan N. Effects on blood pressure of drinking green and black tea. *J Hypertens.* 1999;17:457–463.
152. Nagao T, Hase T, Tokimitsu I. A green tea extract high in catechins reduces body fat and cardiovascular risks in humans. *Obesity (Silver Spring).* 2007;15:1473–1483.
153. Hodgson JM, Devine A, Puddey IB, Chan SY, Beilin LJ, Prince RL. Tea intake is inversely related to blood pressure in older women. *J Nutr.* 2003;133:2883–2886.
154. Lorenz M, Urban J, Engelhardt U, Baumann G, Stangl K, Stangl V. Green and black tea are equally potent stimuli of NO production and vasodilation: New insights into tea ingredients involved. *Basic Res Cardiol.* 2009;104:100–110.
155. Lorenz M, Wessler S, Follmann E, et al. A constituent of green tea, epigallocatechin-3-gallate, activates endothelial nitric oxide synthase by a phosphatidylinositol-3-OH-kinase-, cAMP-dependent protein kinase-, and Akt-dependent pathway and leads to endothelial-dependent vasorelaxation. *J Biol Chem.* 2004;279:6190–6195.
156. Actis-Goretta L, Ottaviani JI, Fraga CG. Inhibition of angiotensin converting enzyme activity by flavanol-rich foods. *J Agric Food Chem.* 2006;54:229–234.
157. Fernández PL, Pablos F, Martín MJ, González AG. Study of catechin and xanthine tea profiles as geographical tracers. *J Agric Food Chem.* 2002;50:1833–1839.
158. Hakim IA, Weisgerber UM, Harris RB, Balentine D, van-Mierlo CAJ, Paetau-Robinson I. Preparation, composition and consumption patterns of tea-based beverages in Arizona. *Nutr Res.* 2000;20:1715–1724.
159. Nakagawa K, Okuda S, Miyazawa T. Dose-dependent incorporation of tea catechins, (-)-epigallocatechin-3-gallate and (-)-epigallocatechin, into human plasma. *Biosci Botechnol Biochem.* 1997;61:1981–1985.
160. Yang CS, Chen L, Lee MJ, Balentine D, Kuo MC, Schantz SP. Blood and urine levels of tea catechins after ingestion of different amounts of green tea by human volunteers. *Cancer Epidemiol Biomarkers Prev.* 1998;7:351–354.

161. St Leger AS, Cochrane AL, Moore F. Factors associated with cardiac mortality in developed countries with particular reference to the consumption of wine. *Lancet*. 1979;1:1017–1020.
162. Doll R, Peto R, Hall E, Wheatley K, Gray R. Mortality in relation to consumption of alcohol: 13 years' observations on male British doctors. *BMJ*. 1994;309:911–918.
163. Gordon T, Kannel WB. Drinking and mortality. The Framingham study. *Am J Epidemiol*. 1984;120:97–107.
164. Gaziano JM, Gaziano TA, Glynn RJ, et al. Light-to-moderate alcohol consumption and mortality in the Physician's Health Study enrollment cohort. *J Am Coll Cardiol*. 2000;35:96–105.
165. Thun MJ, Peto R, Lopez AD, et al. Alcohol consumption and mortality among middle-aged and elderly U.S. adults. *N Engl J Med*. 1997;337:1705–1714.
166. Suh I, Shaten BJ, Cutler JA, Kuller LH. Alcohol use and mortality from coronary heart disease: The role of high-density lipoprotein cholesterol. *Ann Intern Med*. 1992;116:881–887.
167. Mukamal KJ, Conigrave KM, Mittleman MA, et al. Roles of drinking pattern and type of alcohol consumed in coronary heart disease in men. *N Engl J Med*. 2003;348:109–118.
168. Di Castelnuovo A, Rotondo S, Iacoviello L, Donati MB, De Gaetano G. Meta-analysis of wine and beer consumption in relation to vascular risk. *Circulation*. 2002;105:2836–2844.
169. Rimm EB, Williams P, Fosher K, Criqui M, Stampfer MJ. Moderate alcohol intake and lower risk of coronary heart disease: Meta-analysis of effects on lipids and haemostatic factors. *BMJ*. 1999;319:1523–1528.
170. Albert CM, Manson JE, Cook NR, Ajani UA, Gaziano JM, Hennekens CH. Moderate alcohol consumption and the risk of sudden cardiac death among U.S. male physicians. *Circulation*. 1999;100:944–950.
171. Mukamal KJ, Chiuve SE, Rimm EB. Alcohol consumption and risk for coronary heart disease in men with healthy lifestyles. *Arch Intern Med*. 2006;166:2145–2150.
172. Camargo CA, Stampfer MJ, Glynn RJ, et al. Moderate alcohol consumption and risk for angina pectoris or myocardial infarction in U.S. male physicians. *Ann Intern Med*. 1997;126:372–375.
173. Teragawa H, Fukuda Y, Matsuda K, et al. Effect of alcohol consumption on endothelial function in men with coronary artery disease. *Atherosclerosis*. 2002;165:145–152.
174. Imhof A, Woodward M, Doering A, et al. Overall alcohol intake, beer, wine, and systemic markers of inflammation in western Europe: Results from three MONICA samples (Augsburg, Glasgow, Lille). *Eur Heart J*. 2004;25:2092–2100.
175. Kloner RA, Rezkalla SH. To drink or not to drink? That is the question. *Circulation*. 2007;116:1306–1317.
176. Shaper AG, Wannamethee G, Whincup P. Alcohol and blood pressure in middle-aged British men. *J Hum Hypertens*. 1988;2:71–78.
177. Klatsky AL, Friedman GD, Armstrong MA. The relationships between alcoholic beverage use and other traits to blood pressure: A new Kaiser Permanente study. *Circulation*. 1986;73:628–636.
178. Paulin JM, Simpson FO, Waal-Manning HJ. Alcohol consumption and blood pressure in a New Zealand community study. *NZ Med J*. 1985;98:425–428.

179. Gillman MW, Cook NR, Evans DA, Rosner B, Hennekens CH. Relationship of alcohol intake with blood pressure in young adults. *Hypertension.* 1995;25:1106–1110.
180. Grogan JR, Kochar MS. Alcohol and hypertension. *Arch Fam Med.* 1994;3:150–154.
181. Grassi GM, Somers VK, Renk WS, Abboud FM, Mark AL. Effects of alcohol intake on blood pressure and sympathetic nerve activity in normotensive humans: A preliminary report. *J Hypertens Suppl.* 1989;7:S20–S21.
182. Ibsen H, Christensen NJ, Rasmussen S, Hollnagel H, Damkjaer Nielsen M, Giese J. The influence of chronic high alcohol intake on blood pressure, plasma noradrenaline concentration and plasma renin concentration. *Clin Sci (Lond).* 1981;61 (suppl 7);377s–379s.
183. Grønbaek M, Becker U, Johansen D. Type of alcohol consumed and mortality from all causes, coronary heart disease, and cancer. *Ann Intern Med.* 2000;133:411–419.
184. Grønbaek M, Deis A, Sørensen TI, Becker U, Schnohr P, Jensen G. Mortality associated with moderate intakes of wine, beer, or spirits. *BMJ.* 1995;310:1165–1169.
185. Ruidavets JB, Bataille V, Dallongeville J, et al. Alcohol intake and diet in France, the prominent role of lifestyle. *Eur Heart J.* 2004;25:1153–1162.
186. Rosell M, De Faire U, Hellénius ML. Low prevalence of the metabolic syndrome in wine drinkers—Is it the alcohol beverage or the lifestyle? *Eur J Clin Nutr.* 2003;57:227–234.
187. Wannamethee SG, Shaper AG. Type of alcoholic drink and risk of major coronary heart disease events and all-cause mortality. *Am J Public Health.* 1999;89:685–690.
188. Schröder H, Ferrández O, Jimenez Conde J, Sánchez-Font A, Marrugat J. Cardiovascular risk profile and type of alcohol beverage consumption: A population-based study. *Ann Nutr Metab.* 2005;49:100–106.
189. Rimm EB, Stampfer MJ. Wine, beer and spirits: Are they really horses of a different color? *Circulation.* 2002;105:2806–2807.
190. van Velden DP, Mansvelt EP, Fourie E, Rossouw M, Marais AD. The cardioprotective effect of wine on human blood chemistry. *Ann NY Acad Sci.* 2002;957:337–340.
191. Porteri E, Rizzoni D, De Ciuceis C, et al. Vasodilator effects of red wines in subcutaneous small resistance artery of patients with essential hypertension. *Am J Hypertens.* 2010;23:373–378.
192. Klatsky AL, Friedman GD, Armstrong MA, Kipp H. Wine, liquor, beer and mortality. *Am J Epidemiol.* 2003;158:585–595.
193. Lekakis J, Rallidis LS, Andreadou I, et al. Polyphenolic compounds from red grapes acutely improve endothelial function in patients with coronary disease. *Eur J Cardiovasc Prev Rehabil.* 2005;12:596–600.
194. Karatzi KN, Papamichael CM, Karatzis EN, et al. Red wine acutely induces favorable effects on wave reflections and central pressures in coronary artery disease patients. *Am J Hypertens.* 2005;18:1161–1167.
195. Serafini M, Maiani G, Ferro-Luzzi A. Alcohol-free red wine enhances plasma antioxidant capacity in humans. *J Nutr.* 1998;128:1003–1007.
196. Stein JH, Keevil JG, Wiebe DA, Aeschlimann S, Folts JD. Purple grape juice improves endothelial function and reduces susceptibility of LDL cholesterol to oxidation in patients with coronary artery disease. *Circulation.* 1999;100:1050–1055.

197. Kerry NL, Abbey M. Red wine and fractionated phenolic compounds prepared from red wine inhibit low density lipoprotein oxidation *in vitro*. *Atherosclerosis*. 1997;135:93–102.
198. Freedman JE, Parker C 3rd, Li L, et al. Select flavonoids and whole juice from purple grapes inhibit platelet function and enhance nitric oxide release. *Circulation*. 2001;103:2792–2798.
199. Keevil JG, Osman HE, Reed JD, Folts JD. Grape juice, but not orange juice or grapefruit juice, inhibits human platelet aggregation. *J Nutr*. 2000;130:53–56.
200. Iijima K, Yoshizumi M, Hashimoto M, et al. Red wine polyphenols inhibit proliferation of vascular smooth muscle cells and downregulate expression of cyclin A gene. *Circulation*. 2000;22:805–811.
201. Ralay Ranaivo H, Diebolt M, Andriantsitohaina R. Wine polyphenols induce hypotension, and decrease cardiac reactivity and infarct size in rats: Involvement of nitric oxide. *Br J Pharmacol*. 2004;142:671–678.
202. Soares De Moura R, Costa Viana FS, Souza MA, et al. Antihypertensive, vasodilator and antioxidant effects of a vinifera grape skin extract. *J Pharm Pharmacol*. 2002;54:1515–1520.
203. Diebolt M, Bucher B, Andriantsitohaina R. Wine polyphenols decrease blood pressure, improve NO vasodilatation, and induce gene expression. *Hypertension*. 2001;38:159–165.
204. Papamichael C, Karatzi K, Karatzis E, et al. Combined acute effects of red wine consumption and cigarette smoking on haemodynamics of young smokers. *J Hypertens*. 2006;24:1287–1292.
205. Foppa M, Fuchs FD, Preissler L, Andrighetto A, Rosito GA, Duncan BB. Red wine with noon meal lowers post-meal blood pressure: A randomized trial in centrally obese, hypertensive patients. *J Stud Alcohol*. 2002;63:247–251.
206. Park YK, Kim JS, Kang MH. Concord grape juice supplementation reduces blood pressure in Korean hypertensive men: Double-blind, placebo controlled intervention trial. *Biofactors*. 2004;22:145–147.
207. Zilkens RR, Burke V, Hodgson JM, Barden A, Beilin LJ, Puddey IB. Red wine and beer elevate blood pressure in normotensive men. *Hypertension*. 2005;45:874–879.
208. van Mierlo LA, Zock PL, van der Knaap HC, Draijer R. Grape polyphenols do not affect vascular function in healthy men. *J Nutr*. 2010;140:1769–1773.
209. Retterstol L, Berge KE, Braaten Ø, Eikvar L, Pedersen TR, Sandvik L. A daily glass of red wine: Does it affect markers of inflammation? *Alcohol Alcohol*. 2005;40:102–105.
210. Wallerath T, Poleo D, Li H, Förstermann U. Red wine increases the expression of human endothelial nitric oxide synthase: A mechanism that may contribute to its beneficial cardiovascular effects. *J Am Coll Cardiol*. 2003;41:471–478.
211. Leikert JF, Räthel TR, Wohlfart P, Cheynier V, Vollmar AM, Dirsch VM. Red wine polyphenols enhance endothelial nitric oxide synthase expression and subsequent nitric oxide release from endothelial cells. *Circulation*. 2002;106:1614–1617.
212. Honsho S, Sugiyama A, Takahara A, Satoh Y, Nakamura Y, Hashimoto K. A red wine vinegar beverage can inhibit the renin-angiotensin system: Experimental evidence *in vivo*. *Biol Pharm Bull*. 2005;28:1208–1210.
213. Liu BL, Zhang X, Zhang W, Zhen HN. New enlightenment of French Paradox: Resveratrol's potential for cancer chemoprevention and anti-cancer therapy. *Cancer Biol Ther*. 2007;6:1833–1836.

214. Leiro J, Arranz JA, Fraiz N, Sanmartín ML, Quezada E, Orallo F. Effect of cis-resveratrol on genes involved in nuclear factor kappa B signaling. *Int Immunopharmacol.* 2005;5:393–406.
215. Leonard SS, Jiang BH, Stinefelt B, et al. Resveratrol scavenges reactive oxygen species and effects radical-induced cellular responses. *Biochem Biophys Res Commun.* 2003;309:1017–1026.
216. Das S, Das DK. Anti-inflammatory responses of resveratrol. *Inflamm Allergy Drug Targets.* 2007;6:168–173.
217. Csiszar A, Smith K, Labinskyy N, Orosz Z, Rivera A, Ungvari Z. Resveratrol attenuates TNF-alpha-induced activation of coronary arterial endothelial cells: Role of NF-kappaB inhibition. *Am J Physiol Heart Circ Physiol.* 2006;29:H1694–H1699.
218. Stef G, Csiszar A, Lerea K, Ungvari Z, Veress G. Resveratrol inhibits aggregation of platelets from high-risk cardiac patients with aspirin resistance. *J Cardiovasc Pharmacol.* 2006;48:1–5.
219. Poussier B, Cordova AC, Becquemin JP, Sumpio BE. Resveratrol inhibits vascular smooth muscle cell proliferation and induces apoptosis. *J Vasc Surg.* 2005;42:1190–1197.
220. Wallerath T, Deckert G, Ternes T, et al. Resveratrol, polyphenolic phytoalexin present in red wine, enhances expression and activity of endothelial nitric oxide synthase. *Circulation.* 2002;106:1652–1658.
221. Takahashi S, Uchiyama T, Toda K. Differential effect of resveratrol on nitric oxide production in endothelial f-2 cells. *Biol Pharm Bull.* 2009;32:1840–1843.
222. Cheng TH, Liu JC, Lin H, et al. Inhibitory effect of resveratrol on angiotensin II-induced cardiomyocyte hypertrophy. *Naunyn Schmiedebergs Arch Pharmacol.* 2004;369:239–244.
223. Ghanim H, Sia CL, Abuaysheh S, et al. An antiinflammatory and reactive oxygen species suppressive effects of an extract of Polygonum cuspidatum containing resveratrol. *J Clin Endocrinol Metab.* 2010;95:E1–8.
224. Wong RH, Howe PR, Buckley JD, Coates AM, Kunz I, Berry NM. Acute resveratrol supplementation improves flow-mediated dilation in overweight/obese individuals with mildly elevated blood pressure. *Nutr Metab Cardiovasc Dis.* 2011 Nov;21(11):851–856.
225. Opie LH, Lecour S. The red wine hypothesis: From concepts to protective signaling molecules. *Eur Heart J.* 2007;28:1683–1693.
226. Goldberg DM, Yan J, Soleas GJ. Absorption of three wine-related polyphenols in three different matrices by healthy people. *Clin Biochem.* 2003;36:79–87.
227. Allard JS, Perez E, Zou S, de Cabo R. Dietary activators of Sirt1. *Mol Cell Endocrinol.* 2009;299:58–63.
228. Baur JA, Pearson KJ, Price NL, et al. Resveratrol improves health and survival of mice on a high-calorie diet. *Nature.* 2006;444:337–342.
229. Sánchez M, Galisteo M, Vera R, et al. Quercetin downregulates NADPH oxidase, increase eNOS activity and prevents endothelial dysfunction in spontaneously hypertensive rats. *J Hyptertens.* 2006;24:75–84.
230. Perez-Vizcaino F, Duarte J, Andriantsitohaina R. Endothelial function and cardiovascular disease: Effects of quercetin and wine polyphenols. *Free Radic Res.* 2006;40:1054–1065.
231. Rivera L, Morón R, Sánchez M, Zarzuelo A, Galisteo M. Quercetin ameliorates metabolic syndrome and improves the inflammatory status in obese Zucker rats. *Obesity (Silver Spring).* 2008;16:2081–2087.

232. Loke WM, Proudfoot JM, McKinley AJ, et al. Quercetin and its *in vivo* metabolites inhibit neutrophil-mediated low-density lipoprotein oxidation. *J Agric Food Chem.* 2008;56:3609–3615.

233. Alcocer F, Whitley D, Salazar-Gonzalez JF, et al. Quercetin inhibits human vascular smooth muscle cell proliferation and migration. *Surgery.* 2002;131:198–204.

234. Perez-Vizcaino F, Duarte J, Jimenez R, Santos-Buelga C, Osuna A. Antihypertensive effects of the flavonoid quercetin. *Pharmacol Rep.* 2009;61:67–75.

235. Edwards RL, Lyon T, Litwin SE, Rabovsky A, Symons JD, Jalili T. Quercetin reduces blood pressure in hypertensive subjects. *J Nutr.* 2007;137:2405–2411.

236. Egert S, Bosy-Westphal A, Seiberl J, et al. Quercetin reduces systolic blood pressure and plasma low-density lipoprotein concentrations in overweight subjects with a high-cardiovascular disease risk phenotype: A double-blinded, placebo-controlled cross-over study. *Br J Nutr.* 2009;102:1065–1074.

237. Häckl LP, Cuttle G, Dovichi SS, Lima-Landman MT, Nicolau M. Inhibition of angiotensin-converting enzyme by quercetin alters vascular response to bradykinin and angiotensin I. *Pharmacology.* 2002;65:182–186.

238. Hayes KC. Taurine requirement in primates. *Nutr Rev.* 1985;43:65–70.

239. Yamori Y, Liu L, Mizushima S, Ikeda K, Nara Y, CARDIAC Study Group. Male cardiovascular mortality and dietary markers in 25 population samples of 16 countries. *J Hypertens.* 2006;24:1499–1505.

240. Yamori Y, Liu L, Ikeda K, et al. Distribution of twenty-four hour urinary taurine excretion and association with ischemic heart disease mortality in 24 populations of 16 countries: Results from the WHO-CARDIAC study. *Hypertens Res.* 2001;24:453–457.

241. Yamori Y, Liu L, Mori M, et al. Taurine as the nutritional factor for the longevity of the Japanese revealed by a world-wide epidemiological survey. *Adv Exp Med Biol.* 2009;643:13–25.

242. Milei J, Ferreira R, Llesuy S, Forcada P, Covarrubias J, Boveris A. Reduction of reperfusion injury with preoperative rapid intravenous infusion of taurine during myocardial revascularization. *Am Heart J.* 1992;123:339–345.

243. Azuma J, Sawamura A, Awata N. Usefulness of taurine in chronic congestive heart failure and its prospective application. *Jpn Circ J.* 1992;56:95-99.

244. Azuma J, Sawamura A, Awata N, et al. Therapeutic effect of taurine in congestive heart failure: A double-blind crossover trial. *Clin Cardiol.* 1985;8:276–282.

245. Jeejeebhoy F, Keith M, Freeman M, et al. Nutritional supplementation with MyoVive repletes essential cardiac myocytes nutrients and reduces left ventricular size in patients with left ventricular dysfunction. *Am Heart J.* 2002;143:1092–1100.

246. Xu YJ, Arneja AS, Tappia PS, Dhalla NS. The potential health benefits of taurine in cardiovascular disease. *Exp Clin Cardiol.* 2008;13:57–65.

247. Kramer JH, Chovan JP, Schaffer SW. Effect of taurine on calcium paradox and ischemic heart failure. *Am J Physiol.* 1981;240:H238–H246.

248. Xu YJ, Arneja AS, Tappia PS, Dhalla NS. MAPK activation and apoptotic alterations in hearts subjected to calcium paradox are attenuated by taurine. *Cardiovasc Res.* 2006;72:163–174.

249. Ishikawa M, Arai S, Takano M, Hamada A, Kunimasa K, Mori M. Taurine's health influence on Japanese high school girls. *J Biomed Sci.* 2010;17(suppl 1):S47.

250. Zhang M, Bi LF, Fang JH, et al. Beneficial effects of taurine on serum lipids in overweight or obese non-diabetic subjects. *Amino Acids.* 2004;26:267–271.

251. Mizushima S, Nara Y, Sawamura M, Yamori Y. Effects of oral taurine supplementation on lipids and sympathetic nerve tone. *Adv Exp Med Biol.* 1996;403:615–622.

252. Murakami S, Kondo Y, Toda Y, et al. Effect of taurine on cholesterol metabolism in hamsters: Up-regulation of low density lipoprotein (LDL) receptor by taurine. *Life Sci.* 2002;70:2335–2366.

253. Kozumbo WJ, Agarwal S, Koren HS. Breakage and binding of DNA by reaction products of hypochlorous acid with aniline, 1-naphthylamine, or 1-naphthol. *Toxicol Appl Pharmacol.* 1992;115:107–115.

254. Schuller-Levis GB, Park E. Taurine and its chloramine: Modulators of immunity. *Neurochem Res.* 2004;29:117–126.

255. Balkan J, Oztezcan S, Hatipoglu A, Cevikbas U, Aykac-Toker G, Uysal M. Effect of taurine treatment on the regression of existing atherosclerotic lesions in rabbits fed on a high-cholesterol diet. *Biosci Biotechnol Biochem.* 2004;68:1035–1039.

256. Moloney MA, Casey RG, O'Donnell DH, Fitzgerald P, Thompson C, Bouchier-Hayes DJ. Two weeks taurine supplementation reverses endothelial dysfunction in young male type 1 diabetics. *Diab Vasc Dis Res.* 2010;7:300–310.

257. Fennessy FM, Moneley DS, Wang JH, Kelly CJ, Bouchier-Hayes DJ. Taurine and vitamin C modify monocyte and endothelial dysfunction in young smokers. *Circulation.* 2003;107:410–415.

258. Franconi F, Bennardini F, Mattana A, et al. Plasma and platelet taurine are reduced in subjects with insulin-dependent diabetes mellitus: Effects of taurine supplementation. *Am J Clin Nutr.* 1995;61:1115–1119.

259. Ozcan U, Yilmaz E, Ozcan L, et al. Chemical chaperones reduce ER stress and restore glucose homeostasis in a mouse model of type 2 diabetes. *Science.* 2006;313:1137–1140.

260. Ogawa M, Takahara A, Ishijima M, Tazaki S. Decrease of plasma sulfur amino acids in essential hypertension. *Jpn Circ J.* 1985;49:1217–1224.

261. Kohashi N, Katori R. Decrease of urinary taurine in essential hypertension. *Jpn Heart J.* 1983;24:91–102.

262. Liu L, Liu L, Ding Y, et al. Ethnic and environmental differences in various markers of dietary intake and blood pressure among Chinese Han and three other minority peoples of China: Results from the WHO Cardiovascular Diseases and Alimentary Comparison (CARDIAC) Study. *Hypertens Res.* 2001;24:315–322.

263. Mizushima S, Moriguchi EH, Ishikawa P, et al. Fish intake and cardiovascular risk among middle-aged Japanese in Japan and Brazil. *J Cardiovasc Risk.* 1997;4:191–199.

264. Fujita T, Ando K, Noda H, Ito Y, Sato Y. Effects of increased adrenomedullary activity and taurine in young patients with borderline hypertension. *Circulation.* 1987;75:525–532.

265. Inoue A, Takahashi H, Lee LC, et al. Retardation of the development of hypertension in DOCA salt rats by taurine supplement. *Cardiovasc Res.* 1998;22:351–358.

266. Sato Y, Ando K, Fujita T. Role of sympathetic nervous system in hypotensive action of taurine in DOCA-salt rats. *Hypertension.* 1987;9:81–87.

267. Ji Y, Tao L, Xu HL, Rao MR. [Effects of taurine and enalapril on blood pressure, platelet aggregation and the regression of left ventricular hypertrophy in two-kidney-one-clip renovascular hypertensive rats]. *Yao Xue Xue Bao.* 1995;30:886–890.

268. Hano T, Kasano M, Tomari H, Iwane N. Taurine suppresses pressor response through the inhibition of sympathetic nerve activity and the improvement in baro-reflex sensitivity of spontaneously hypertensive rats. *Adv Exp Med Biol.* 2009;643:57–63.

269. Trachtman H, Del Pizzo R, Rao P, Rujikarn N, Sturman JA. Taurine lowers blood pressure in the spontaneously hypertensive rat by a catecholamine independent mechanism. *Am J Hypertens.* 1989;2(12 Pt 1):909–912.

270. Hu J, Xu X, Yang J, Wu G, Sun C, Lv Q. Antihypertensive effect of taurine in rat. *Adv Exp Med Biol.* 2009;643:75–84.

271. Yamamoto J, Akabane S, Yoshimi H, Nakai M, Ikeda M. Effects of taurine on stress-evoked hemodynamic and plasma catecholamine changes in spontaneously hypertensive rats. *Hypertension.* 1985;7(6 Pt 1):913–922.

272. Fujita T, Sato Y. Hypotensive effect of taurine. Possible involvement of the sympathetic nervous system and endogenous opiates. *J Clin Invest.* 1988;82:993–997.

273. Kong WX, Chen SW, Li YL, et al. Effects of taurine on rat behaviors in three anxiety models. *Pharmacol Biochem Behav.* 2006;83:271–276.

274. Schaffer SW, Lombardini JB, Azuma J. Interaction between the actions of taurine and angiotensin II. *Amino Acids.* 2000;18:305–318.

275. Nandhini AR, Anuradha CV. Hoe 140 abolishes the blood pressure lowering effect of taurine in high fructose-fed rats. *Amino Acids.* 2004;26:299–303.

276. Shao A, Hathcock JN. Risk assessment for the amino acids taurine, L-glutamine and L-arginine. *Regul Toxicol Pharmacol.* 2008;50:376–399.

277. Wollin SD, Jones PJ. Alpha-lipoic acid and cardiovascular disease. *J Nutr.* 2003;133:3327–3330.

278. Packer L, Witt EH, Tritschler HJ. Alpha-lipoic acid as a biological antioxidant. *Free Radic Biol Med.* 1995;19:227–250.

279. Sola S, Mir MQ, Cheema FA, et al. Irbesartan and lipoic acid improve endothelial function and reduce markers of inflammation in the metabolic syndrome: Results of the Irbesartan and Lipoic Acid in Endothelial Dysfunction (ISLAND) study. *Circulation.* 2005;111:343–348.

280. Zulkhairi A, Zaiton Z, Jamaluddin M, et al. Alpha lipoic acid possess dual antioxidant and lipid lowering properties in atherosclerotic-induced New Zealand white rabbit. *Biomed Pharmacother.* 2008;62:716–722.

281. Kamenova P. Improvement of insulin sensitivity in patients with type 2 diabetes mellitus after oral administration of alpha-lipoic acid. *Hormones (Athens).* 2006;5:251–258.

282. Jacob S, Zaiton Z, Jamaluddin M, et al. Oral administration of RAC-alpha-lipoic acid modulates insulin sensitivity in patients with type-2-diabetes mellitus: A placebo-controlled pilot trial. *Free Radic Biol Med.* 1999;27:309–314.

283. Konrad T, Vicini P, Kusterer K, et al. alpha-Lipoic acid treatment decreases serum lactate and pyruvate concentrations and improves glucose effectiveness in lean and obese patients with type 2 diabetes. *Diabetes Care.* 1999;22:280–287.

284. Estrada DE, Ewart HS, Tsakiridis T, et al. Stimulation of glucose uptake by the natural coenzyme alpha-lipoic acid/thioctic acid: Participation of elements of the insulin signaling pathway. *Diabetes.* 1996;45:1798–1804.

285. Ziegler D, Ametov A, Barinov A, et al. Oral treatment with α-lipoic acid improves symptomatic diabetic polyneuropathy. The SYDNEY 2 trial. *Diabetes Care.* 2006;29:2365–2370.

286. Tankova T, Cherninkova S, Koev D. Treatment for diabetic mononeuropathy with alpha-lipoic acid. *Int J Clin Pract.* 2005;59:645–650.

287. Ziegler D, Hanefeld M, Ruhnau KJ, et al. Treatment of symptomatic diabetic peripheral neuropathy with the anti-oxidant alpha-lipoic acid. A 3-week multicenter randomized controlled trial (ALADIN Study). *Diabetologia* 1995;38:1425–1433.

288. Ziegler D, Nowak H, Kempler P, Vargha P, Low PA. Treatment of symptomatic diabetic polyneuropathy with the antioxidant alpha-lipoic acid: A meta-analysis. *Diabet Med.* 2004;21:114–121.

289. Ziegler D, Schatz H, Conrad F, Gries FA, Ulrich H, Reichel G. Effects of treatment with antioxidant alpha-lipoic acid on cardiac autonomic neuropathy in NIDDM patients. A 4-month randomized controlled multicenter trial (DEKAN Study). Deutsche Kardiale Autonome Neuropathie. *Diabetes Care.* 1997;20:369–373.

290. Vasdev S, Gill V, Parai S, Gadag V. Dietary lipoic acid supplementation attenuates hypertension in Dahl salt sensitive rats. *Mol Cell Biochem.* 2005;275:135–141.

291. Midaoui AE, Elimadi A, Wu L, Haddad PS, de Champlain J. Lipoic acid prevents hypertension, hyperglycemia, and the increase in heart mitochondrial superoxide production. *Am J Hypertens.* 2003;16:173–179.

292. Vasdev S, Ford CA, Parai S, Longerich L, Gadag V. Dietary alpha-lipoic acid supplementation lowers blood pressure in spontaneously hypertensive rats. *J Hypertens.* 2000;18:567–573.

293. Vasdev S, Ford CA, Parai S, Longerich L, Gadag V. Dietary lipoic acid supplementation prevents fructose-induced hypertension in rats. *Nutr Metab Cardiovasc Dis.* 2000;10:339–346.

294. Koçak G, Aktan F, Canbolat O, et al. Alpha-lipoic acid treatment ameliorates metabolic parameters, blood pressure, vascular reactivity and morphology of vessels already damaged by streptozotocin-diabetes. *Diabetes Nutr Metab.* 2000;13:308–318.

295. McMackin CJ, Widlansky ME, Hamburg NM, et al. Effect of combined treatment with alpha-Lipoic acid and acetyl-L-carnitine on vascular function and blood pressure in coronary artery disease patients. *J Clin Hypertens. (Greenwich).* 2007;9:249–255.

296. Takaoka M, Kobayashi Y, Yuba M, Ohkita M, Matsumura Y. Effects of alpha-lipoic acid on deoxycorticosterone acetate-salt-induced hypertension in rats. *Eur J Pharmacol.* 2001;424:121–129.

297. Singh U, Jialal I. Alpha-lipoic acid supplementation and diabetes. *Nutr Rev.* 2008;66:646–657.

chapter nine

Treating hypertension

Blood pressure goals

The first step in treating hypertension is to assign a target or goal blood pressure to the patient. This is a complex task because the various guidelines suggest different values. Furthermore, blood pressure norms change within each guideline depending on the published version and on comorbid conditions (i.e., diabetes or kidney disease). Two well-accepted guidelines are from the Joint National Committee on Prevention, Detection, Evaluation, and Treatment of High Blood Pressure from the United States (JNC 7)[1]; and the Task Force for the Management of Arterial Hypertension of the European Society of Hypertension (ESH) and of the European Society of Cardiology (ESC).[2] The JNC 7 is more simple and direct, although the ESH/ESC, which more meticulously defines cardiovascular risk, is better tailored to the individual despite being more complex. Both recent guidelines suggest lowering office blood pressure to <140/90 mm Hg in otherwise healthy adults, but to <130/80 mm Hg in those with diabetes, renal disease, or cardiovascular disease. However, as white-coat hypertension and white-coat effect are quite common, affecting up to 20% of people with elevated blood pressure,[3] the use of out-of-office measurements with ambulatory or home blood pressure devices is also suggested. Out-of-office blood pressure monitoring is shown to more accurately predict cardiovascular risk[2] and these techniques are gaining popularity. Home blood pressure monitoring is the preferred method in my practice, because it further engages my patients in their care. However, it is used with caution by suggesting only proper and validated devices and avoiding use in people with arrhythmias, as these devices may then be inaccurate. Although not absolutely necessary, it is good practice to check the home blood pressure monitor against an in-office measurement prior to use and periodically thereafter. The 24-hour ambulatory device is also useful because it records values during sleep, which is an important component in ascertaining the cardiovascular risk. However, it is expensive, often not covered by medical insurance, and only represents one day of a person's life. Most blood pressure guidelines suggest comparative values for out-of-office devices

Table 9.1 Guideline Blood Pressure Goals

Source	Office blood pressure (mm Hg)	Ambulatory blood pressure (mm Hg)	Home blood pressure (mm Hg)
Joint National Committee (JNC 7) (2003)	<140/90; But for diabetes, chronic kidney disease, or cardiovascular disease <130/80	< 135/85 while awake; Less than 120/75 during sleep	<130/80
European Society Hypertension/ European Society Cardiology (2007)	<140/90; But for diabetes, chronic kidney disease, or cardiovascular disease <130/80	<125–130/80 over 24 hours <130–135/85 during daytime <120/70 during nighttime	<130–135/85

with in-office values. Table 9.1 outlines the various blood pressure goals for the JNC 7 and the more recent ESH/ESC guidelines.

Out-of-office blood pressure goals for special populations, such as individuals with diabetes and chronic kidney disease, are not as clearly defined. This is unfortunate because these people are at increased risk of cardiovascular and renal disease development and progression. Many studies also suggest a better correlation between cardiovascular disease and out-of-office measurements than with office measurements.[4–8] A few independent studies suggest comparable blood pressure goals to otherwise healthy people, although there is no clear consensus on these values. In those with diabetes, a daytime ambulatory blood pressure of <130/80 mm Hg or a 5–10 mm Hg decrease from the standard nondiabetic values has been suggested.[9,10] In chronic kidney disease, ambulatory blood pressures of <125/75 mm Hg over 24 hours, <130/85 mm Hg during daytime, and <110/70 mm Hg during nighttime have been proposed[11]; others suggest <140/80 mm Hg.[12] Although each study bases its conclusions on valid observations, it is not reasonable to ascribe less stringent blood pressure goals for these special populations compared with standard office goals, which is typically <130/80 mm Hg. A reasonable approach is outlined in Table 9.2, which includes blood pressure goals for most populations with use of all measurement modalities. These values will undoubtedly change over time.

Most guidelines define the inclusion criteria for these special populations. These factors can be easily obtained with a careful history and physical exam, an EKG, and appropriate blood and urine testing. The ESH/ESC guideline provides reasonable definitions as outlined in Table 9.3.

Table 9.2 Reasonable Blood Pressure Goals

Office blood pressure (mm Hg)	Ambulatory blood pressure (mm Hg)	Home blood pressure (mm Hg)
<140/90; For diabetes, chronic kidney disease, or cardiovascular disease <130/80	<130/80 over 24 hours <135/85 during daytime <120/70 during nighttime For diabetes, chronic kidney disease, or cardiovascular disease <125/75 over 24 hours, <130/80 during daytime, <110/70 during nighttime	<135/85; For diabetes, chronic kidney disease, or cardiovascular disease <130/80

Table 9.3 Special Populations

Diabetes	Chronic kidney disease	Cardiovascular disease
Fasting plasma glucose ≥126 mg/dL	Diabetic nephropathy	Myocardial infarction, angina, heart failure, coronary revascularization
Postload plasma glucose ≥198 mg/dL	Serum creatinine (M >1.5; F >1.4 mg/dL)	Ischemic stroke, cerebral hemorrhage, TIA
	Proteinuria (>300 mg/24 hr)	Peripheral artery disease
		Retinopathy

The tables for blood pressure goals and definitions of special populations can also be found in Appendix C.

Approach to treating hypertension

Prior to studying medicine and becoming a physician, I had the opportunity to do research at an elite academic institution. Although I still consider myself a scientist, I truly brandished this title at that time. Two principles, perhaps even axioms, became apparent during my studies. The first is that the truth is always simple. My research was mostly in the field of physics, as I studied the energy levels of small hydrocarbon radicals in ultrahigh vacuum chambers. In fact, the astrophysics community was most interested in my work. This research was quite repetitive and complex, requiring years of allocated effort. However, when proper energy spectra were obtained, the corresponding analysis was always a simple fit. Despite often tedious pursuit in incorrectly explaining the data, the final true analysis was always simple and mostly corroborated my initial expectations. The second principle is that synergy—combining two or more forces to yield a product larger than the sum of its individual parts—is a powerful tool. With synergy, one plus one does not always equal two but can be three or more. Although my research was clearly in the field of physics, my doctorate was in chemistry. By combining knowledge from both disciplines, I was able to generate elusive radical molecules that were once thought impossible to study. Through synergy, I was able to achieve impressive results. I have applied these two principles to my study and practice of medicine as well. For example, if a diagnosis is too complex I often reconsider because it is often wrong. Treatment of illness is also best approached in a simple and direct way and hypertension is no exception. The field of medicine and hypertension, in particular, is greatly indebted to the work of Dr. John Laragh and his colleagues. Through many decades of research, they defined the mechanics of blood pressure support and hypertension, and designed simple schemes or algorithms to treat the disease. Their method—called the Laragh method—allows a simple characterization of the etiology of hypertension, and then proposes the most direct treatment course using the fewest medicines possible. The approach is intelligent, as opposed to the random stab at treatment with a physician's most-favored medicine, and should guide adequate therapy with a quicker response and fewer drugs. Its efficacy is shown compared with standard treatment by clinical hypertension specialists.[13] It is outlined in a series of review articles in the *American Journal of Hypertension* in 2001[14] and more recently modified.[15] Laragh describes blood pressure in terms of two supporting systems. The primary system is the volume or salt/water mediated system which supports a normal and sometimes abnormal blood pressure. However, if an individual is salt/water depleted as may occur with dehydration, either from natural or medicinal causes, the renin–angiotensin–aldosterone system (RAAS) is activated as a backup support to the blood pressure. In this way, these two systems act in concert, where if adequate salt/water/volume is present and if the blood pressure is normal, the RAAS is turned off. As hypertension is a disease state, these two systems often act independently, and states of either elevated volume, abnormal renin–angiotensin–aldosterone activity, or a combination can occur. The Laragh method, with the assistance of an algorithm, helps characterize the type of hypertension and then its simplest course of treatment. It carefully defines each class of antihypertensive medication into either an anti-renin–angiotensin system agent (R-type) or an antivolume agent (V-type). Through measurement of the plasma renin activity (PRA), which is a proxy for the entire RAAS, the cause of hypertension can be determined. For example if the PRA is ≥0.65 ng/mL/hr, which is considered the cutoff for significant participation of the RAAS in hypertension, a person would benefit from an R-type medication. If the PRA is <0.65 ng/mL/hr, a V-type medicine should be initiated. Repeat PRA testing is subsequently used to guide further management. The PRA is also useful in screening for renovascular disease as a value >1.6 ng/mL/hr makes this diagnosis more likely, and if the PRA is low and the serum aldosterone level is inappropriately elevated, an adrenal/aldosterone (i.e. hyperadrenal) mediated cause must be considered. The Endocrine Society of the United States provides rather vague guidelines, but suggests further evaluation for primary aldosteronism in people with hypertension and the following: a low PRA, a high plasma aldosterone concentration (PAC) (>15 ng/dL), and a PAC/PRA ratio of 20 and above.[16] As both of these causes are potentially treated and cured with surgical intervention, a nonmedicinal treatment must be considered and referral to a hypertension specialist is advised. The Laragh method can be applied to individuals not yet taking medication as well as to those already undergoing treatment. Overall, this classification and approach to treating hypertension is simple and easily applied, which likely portends to its truth.

An interesting deviation of the Laragh method, from most standard approaches and algorithms in treating hypertension, is its ability and emphasis on subtracting nonessential medications. Certainly, fewer medicines will reduce the cost of treatment and improve patient compliance. Imagine the delighted smile on a patient's face when told that in treating their hypertension a medicine should be stopped. However, reduction of nonessential medications may have far more important implications, not only in better managing hypertension but in reducing risk of cardiovascular events. Paradoxical increases in blood pressure with initiation of medicines is well described.[17,18] Even standard lifestyle modifications, such as reduction in salt intake, may cause an increase in blood pressure in some people.[19] With use of V-type medicines, the explanation for this effect may be from further induction of the RAAS, especially in those who already have elevated PRA. High-renin hypertension will only minimally respond to contraction of the blood plasma compartment, but a significantly greater pressor effect from angiotensin II may occur, causing further increase in blood pressure. For R-type medicines, this effect occurs in those with low PRA levels, possibly due to unopposed α-adrenergic activity without a compensatory decrease in blood pressure, as the medicine has only limited ability to act. Furthermore, elevated PRA levels are associated with cardiovascular disease,[20] presumably as they are a proxy for the entire RAAS. Guidance of hypertension management with PRA levels, as suggested by the Laragh method, should obviate these pitfalls.

The British Hypertension Society also considers the activity of the RAAS in its approach to hypertension treatment.[21] Although it doesn't suggest initial measurement of the PRA, it does use renin profiling. For example, if a person with hypertension is young (i.e., <55 years) and not black, then an R-type medication is started because renin-mediated hypertension is more common in this population. For older or black people with hypertension, who more commonly have volume-mediated hypertension, a V-type medication is first prescribed. If a second medicine is needed, a complementary type is added. Their scheme is often referred to as the "AB/CD" method, where A represents angiotensin-converting enzyme inhibitors and angiotensin receptor blockers, B the beta blockers, C the calcium channel blockers, and D the diuretics. If a third medicine is needed, the society suggests adding a V-type medicine (i.e., C or D), as the RAAS has already been blocked. A later amendment discourages use of beta blockers in the primary treatment of hypertension, because they may be associated with insulin insensitivity and diabetes, although the society recognizes their importance in treating heart disease.[22] As such, the scheme may be more appropriately called the "A/CD" method. This approach is also intelligent and minimizes use of medication.

Throughout this book, various natural or holistic techniques of lowering blood pressure have been described, each of which has been characterized in terms of its R-type and V-type properties. For example, physical activity is a V-type method, whereas vitamin D supplementation is an R-type method. As less scientific data is available in both biological and clinical characterization of these techniques, it is more difficult to clearly define these properties. Sometimes a combination of both types is ascribed, as it is difficult to determine if one component outweighs the other. Yet, it is a reasonably accurate characterization of these natural and holistic approaches. Appendix A lists these methods and also includes standard medications such as diuretics and beta blockers. Appendix B provides more detail about specific dosing and the efficacy of the various techniques. Incorporation of these techniques into established methods, such as those just described, affords a unique way of treating hypertension. It allows a truly holistic approach in that it involves all aspects of a person's life from medicine, to diet, to physical activity. My experience with such an approach has been positive, as my patients have become more engaged in their overall health. Of course, everyone has limitations in the extent of their adherence, whether dietary or medicinal, but it is easier for them to meet their goals when offered a broader variety of options. The synergy of these two approaches, that is, the pharmaceutical and the natural, allows for a truly holistic and more powerful way of treating hypertension.

References

1. Chobanian AV, Bakris GL, Black HR, et al. Seventh Report of the Joint National Committee on Prevention, Detection, Evaluation, and Treatment of High Blood Pressure. *Hypertension.* 2003;42:1206–1252.
2. Mancia G, De Backer G, Dominiczak A, et al. 2007 Guidelines for management of arterial hypertension: The Task Force for the Management of Arterial Hypertension of the European Society of Hypertension (ESH) and of the European Society of Cardiology (ESC). *Eur Heart J.* 2007;28:1462–1536.
3. Pickering TG, James GD, Boddie C, Harshfield GA, Blank S, Laragh JH. How common is white coat hypertension? *JAMA.* 1988;259:225–228.
4. Kamoi K, Ito T, Miyakoshi M, Minagawa S. Usefulness of home blood pressure measurement in the morning in patients with type 2 diabetes: Long-term results of a prospective longitudinal study. *Clin Exp Hypertens.* 2010;32:184–192.
5. Eguchi K, Pickering TG, Hoshide S, et al. Ambulatory blood pressure is a better marker than clinic blood pressure in predicting cardiovascular events in patients with/without type 2 diabetes. *Am J Hypertens.* 2008;21:443–450.
6. Leitão CB, Canani LH, Silveiro SP, Gross JL. Ambulatory blood pressure monitoring and type 2 diabetes. *Arq Bras Cardiol.* 2007;89:315–321.
7. Minutolo R, Agarwal R, Borrelli S, et al. Prognostic role of ambulatory blood pressure measurement in patients with nondialysis chronic kidney disease. *Arch Intern Med.* 2011;171:1090–1098.
8. Agarwal R. Home and ambulatory blood pressure monitoring in chronic kidney disease. *Curr Opin Nephrol Hypertens.* 2009;18:507–512.
9. Leitão CB, Rodrigues TC, Kramer CK, et al. Which patients with diabetes should undergo ambulatory blood pressure monitoring? *J Hypertens.* 2011;29:236–241.
10. Parati G, Bilo G. Should 24-hour ambulatory blood pressure monitoring be done in every patient with diabetes? *Diabetes Care.* 2009;32(suppl 2):S298–S304.
11. Agarwal R. Ambulatory blood pressure and cardiovascular events in chronic kidney disease. *Semin Nephrol.* 2007;27:538–543.
12. Andersen MJ, Khawandi W, Agarwal R. Home blood pressure monitoring in CKD. *Am J Kidney Dis.* 2005;45:994–1001.
13. Egan BM, Basile JN, Rehman SU, et al. Plasma renin test-guided drug treatment algorithm for correcting patients with treated but uncontrolled hypertension: A randomized controlled trial. *Am J Hypertens.* 2009;22:792–801.
14. Laragh J. Laragh's lessons in pathophysiology and clinical pearls for treating hypertension. *Am J Hypertens.* 2001;14(9 Pt 1):84–89.
15. Laragh JH, Sealey JE. The plasma renin test reveals the contribution of body sodium-volume content(V) and renin-angiotensin (R) vasoconstriction to long-term blood pressure. *Am J Hypertens.* 2011;24:1164–1180.
16. Funder JW, Carey RM, Fardella C, et al. Case detection, diagnosis, and treatment of patients with primary aldosteronism: An endocrine society clinical practice guideline. *J Clin Endocrinol Metab.* 2008;93:3266–3281.
17. Alderman MH, Cohen HW, Sealey JE, Laragh JH. Pressor responses to antihypertensive drug types. *Am J Hypertens.* 2010;23:1031–1037.

18. Drayer JI, Keim HJ, Weber MA, Case DB, Laragh JH. Unexpected pressor responses to propanolol in essential hypertension. An interaction between enini, aldosterone and sympathetic activity. *Am J Med.* 1976;60:897–903.
19. Longworth DL, Drayer JI, Weber MA, Laragh JH. Divergent blood pressure responses during short-term sodium restriction in hypertension. *Clin Pharmacol Ther.* 1980;27:544–546.
20. Gonzalez MC, Cohen HW, Sealey JE, Laragh JH, Alderman MH. Enduring direct association of baseline plasma renin activity with all-cause and cardiovascular mortality in hypertensive patients. *Am J Hypertens.* 2011;24:1181–1186.
21. Williams B, Poulter NR, Brown MJ, et al. Guidelines for management of hypertension: Report of the Fourth Working Party of the British Hypertension Society, 2004-BHS IV. *J Hum Hypertens.* 2004;18:139–185.
22. Sever P. New hypertension guidelines from the National Institute for Health and Clinical Excellence and the British Hypertension Society. *J Renin Angiotensin Aldosterone Syst.* 2006;7:61–63.

Appendix A: Antihypertensive methods

	Type of Antihypertensive	
R (renin)	Mixed	V (volume)
Medications		
		Diuretics
		Calcium channel blockers
		Alpha blockers
		Direct vasodilators
Angiotensin converting enzyme inhibitors		
Angiotensin II receptor blockers		
Direct renin inhibitors		
Beta blockers		
Central alpha agonists		
Diet		
	High potassium diet	Low sodium diet
		High magnesium diet
		Vitamin C supplements
		Folic acid supplements
High calcium diet		
Vitamin D supplements		

High fiber diet

Omega-3 polyunsaturated fats

Low carbohydrate diet

High protein diet

Nonpharmacologic Techniques

Relaxation therapy

Physical activity

Natural Medications

Garlic

L-arginine

Coenzyme Q_{10}

Resveratrol, quercetin, red wine extract

Cocoa powder (some R effect too)

Taurine

Alpha-lipoic acid

Appendix B: Antihypertensive dosing

Antihypertensive dose (adults)

Medications

Diuretics: Hydrochlorothiazide, chlorothiazide, furosemide, torsemide, spironolactone, eplerenone

Calcium channel blockers: Amlodipine, felodipine, nifedipine, diltiazem, verapamil

Alpha blockers: Doxazosin, prazosin, terazosin

Direct vasodilators: Hydralazine, minoxidil, nitrates

Angiotensin converting enzyme inhibitors: Captopril, enalapril, benazepril, fosinopril, lisinopril, ramipril, trandolapril, quinapril

Angiotensin II receptor blockers: Candesartan, irbesartan, losartan, olmesartan, telmisartan, valsartan

Direct renin inhibitors: Aliskiren

Beta blockers: Atenolol, bisoprolol, carvedilol, labetalol, metoprolol, propanolol

Central alpha agonists: Clonidine, methyldopa

Diet

Low sodium diet: Up to 1500 mg/day

High potassium diet: 4700 mg/day or higher

High calcium diet

- Women: 1000 mg/day or higher (up to 50 years), 1200 mg/day or higher (over 50 years)

Antihypertensive dose (adults)

- Men: 1000 mg/day or higher (up to 70 years), 1200 mg/day or higher (over 70 years)

High magnesium diet
- Women: 320 mg/day or higher
- Men: 420 mg/day or higher

Vitamin D: Maintain blood level of 30-49 ng/ml

Vitamin C: Daily supplement of 500 mg/day

Folic acid: Daily supplement of 400 mcg/day

High fiber diet (typical consumption)
- Women: 25 g/day or higher (up to 50 years), 21 g/day or higher (over 50 years)
- Men: 38 g/day or higher (up to 50 years), 30 g/day or higher (over 50 years)

Dietary fats: 20%–35% of total calorie intake
- Minimize trans and saturated fats, increase monounsaturated (and polyunsaturated fats)
- 2 g of OTC fish oil or 1 g of lovaza or 2 to 3 fatty fish meals each week

Carbohydrates: 45%–65% of total calorie intake, should target 45%; favor low glycemic index foods; favor healthy/natural foods (i.e., fruits, vegetables, whole grains)

Proteins: 10%–35% of total calorie intake, should target 35%; favor vegetable protein sources

Nonpharmacologic Techniques

Physical activity: At least 150 minutes of moderate-intensity aerobic activity each week or 75 minutes of vigorous-intensity aerobic activity each week (counts as twice moderate-activity) or combination of both

Relaxation therapy: The Resperate device on most days of the week

Natural Medications

L-arginine: 3 tablets of sustained release (350 mg each tablet) twice daily

Coenzyme Q_{10}: 1 tablet of 100 mg daily (preferably Q-gel preparation)

Garlic: Raw garlic 4 grams (1 to 2 cloves) daily or dried powder (1.3 percent alliin) 300 mg 3 times daily or aged garlic 7.2 grams daily

Cocoa powder: One serving twice daily (high-end, unprocessed brand)

Red wine: Red wine itself does not lower blood pressure; red wine polyphenols (extracts) such as resveratrol and quercitin may lower blood pressure but the supporting evidence is limited; resveratrol 40 mg to 500 mg daily; quercitin 250 mg to 750 mg daily (can be in divided dose twice daily)

Taurine: 1 tablet of 500 mg twice daily

Alpha-lipoic acid: 600 mg once daily (but very limited evidence)

Appendix C: Blood pressure goals and special populations

Blood Pressure Goals

Office blood pressure (mm Hg)	Ambulatory blood pressure (mm Hg)	Home blood pressure (mm Hg)
Less than 140/90	Less than 130/80 over 24 hours, less than 135/85 during daytime, less than 120/70 during nighttime	Less than 135/85
For diabetes, chronic kidney disease, or cardiovascular disease less than 130/80		For diabetes, chronic kidney disease, or cardiovascular disease less than 130/80
	For diabetes, chronic kidney disease or cardiovascular disease less than 125/75 over 24 hours, less than 130/80 during daytime, less than 110/70 during nighttime	

Special Population Criteria		
Diabetes	**Chronic kidney disease**	**Cardiovascular disease**
Fasting plasma glucose ≥126 mg/dL	Diabetic nephropathy	Myocardial infarction, angina, heart failure, coronary revascularization
Postload plasma glucose ≥ 198 mg/dL	Serum creatinine (M >1.5; F >1.4 mg/dL)	Ischemic stroke, cerebral hemorrhage, transient ischemic attack (TIA)
	Proteinuria (>300 mg/24hr)	Peripheral artery disease
		Retinopathy

Index